# MULTIPLE CHOICE QUESTIONS IN GYNAECOLOGY AND OBSTETRICS

# MULTIPLE CHOICE QUESTIONS IN GYNAECOLOGY AND OBSTETRICS

## Third Edition

**Marcus E Setchell** MA, FRCS, FRCOG
Consultant, Department of Obstetrics and Gynaecology, St Bartholomew's
and Homerton Hospitals, London

### and

**Richard J Lilford** PhD, MRCP, FRCOG
Professor of Health Services Research, University of Birmingham

A member of the Hodder Headline Group
LONDON • SYDNEY • AUCKLAND
Co-published in the USA by Oxford University Press, Inc., New York

First published in Great Britain in 1985
Third edition published in 1996
Arnold, a member of the Hodder Headline Group,
338 Euston Road, London NW1 3BH

Co-published in the United States of America by
Oxford University Press, Inc.,
198 Madison Avenue, New York, NY 10016
Oxford is a registered trademark of Oxford University Press

Whilst the advice and information in this book is
believed to be true and accurate at the date of going
to press, neither the authors nor the publisher can
accept any responsibility or liability for any errors or
omissions that may be made. In particular (but
without limiting the generality of the preceding
disclaimer) every effort has been made to check drug
dosages; however, it is still possible that errors have
been missed. Furthermore, dosage schedules are
constantly being revised and new side effects
recognized. For these reasons the reader is strongly
urged to consult the drug companies' printed
instructions before administering any of the drugs
recommended in this book.

*British Library Cataloguing in Publication Data*
A catalogue record for this book is available from the British Library

*Library of Congress Cataloging-in-Publication Data*
A catalog record for this book is available from the Library of Congress

ISBN 0 340 58896 9

Typeset in Garamond and Helvetica
Produced by Gray Publishing, Tunbridge Wells
Printed and bound in Great Britain by J W Arrowsmith Ltd, Bristol

# CONTENTS

# PREFACE

Multiple choice questions are now a standard part of most undergraduate and postgraduate examinations. They are also frequently used as in-course or end-of-course assessments of both learning and teaching.

As with any kind of examinations, practice with the technique may improve performance and enhance confidence. The questions in this book are not intended primarily as examination practice, but rather for students to assess their comprehension and learning of the obstetric and gynaecological course, and particularly their reading of *Ten Teachers*. The answer to virtually every question is to be found in the sixteenth edition of the companion books, *Gynaecology by Ten Teachers* (G) and *Obstetrics by Ten Teachers* (OB), but not always on a single page! The chapter references for each question are to be found on the answer page. The association with *Ten Teachers* does not preclude its usefulness to students who wish to assess their knowledge obtained from other sources. We hope that students will find it helpful to familiarize themselves with MCQs and be encouraged to pace themselves appropriately for examination conditions.

The subject of obstetrics and gynaecology remains part science and part art, and the existence of shades of opinion makes the setting of factual and objective questions particularly difficult. This new edition has undergone expansion and revision, and we have tried to include more explanations about the answers.

We are grateful to the authors of *Ten Teachers*, many of whom have contributed questions to this new edition, to Catherine Walker of Arnold Publishers for helpful suggestions, and to my secretary, Carol Whitehead, for painstaking preparation of the manuscript.

Marcus E Setchell and Richard J Lilford

# PART I

# GYNAECOLOGY

# GYNAECOLOGY

1 The nerve supply to the vulva is derived from:
   (a) The pudendal nerve
   (b) The ilio-inguinal nerve
   (c) The genitofemoral nerve
   (d) The posterior cutaneous nerve of the thigh
   (e) The inferior haemorrhoidal nerve


2 The support of the uterus is provided by:
   (a) The cardinal ligaments
   (b) The round ligaments
   (c) The utero-sacral ligaments
   (d) The integrity of the perineal body
   (e) The broad ligament


3 Menstruation:
   (a) Is not normally accompanied by pain
   (b) Contains blood, mucus and the unfertilized ovum
   (c) The normal range of blood loss is 20–80 ml
   (d) Usually ceases before the age of 48 years
   (e) Is often followed by fluid retention


4 In the menstrual cycle, ovulation:
   (a) Occurs two days after the peak of luteinizing hormone (LH)
   (b) Occurs 14 days before the onset of the menstrual flow
   (c) Occurs when progesterone secretion is at its maximum
   (d) Will only occur as a reflex response to orgasm
   (e) May be inhibited by emotional disturbance


5 After the menopause:
   (a) There is a reduction in vaginal acidity
   (b) Gonadotrophin secretion falls
   (c) Any vaginal bleeding should be investigated by an endometrial biopsy/
       D & C
   (d) Treatment with oestrogen is often beneficial
   (e) The rate of bone loss is greatest in the first two years

**1 (a) True** The pudendal nerve (S2,3,4) gives off the inferior rectal branch before dividing into perineal nerve and dorsal nerve of the clitoris.

**(b) True** The ilio-inguinal and genitofemoral nerves supply sensory fibres
**(c) True** to the mons and labia.

**(d) True** It carries some sensory fibres to the perineum.
**(e) False** This branch of the pudendal nerve supplies the anus and perianal skin

G 1

**2 (a) True** These ligaments are condensations of the visceral pelvic fascia and are the main supports of the uterus and upper vagina.
**(b) False** The round ligament may prevent retroversion, but does not support the uterus.
**(c) True** These condensations of fascia support the cervix.
**(d) False** Unrepaired third degree tear does not lead to uterine prolapse.
**(e) False** This is a peritoneal fold and contains no supportive tissue.

G 1

**3 (a) False** Dysmenorrhoea may occur physiologically especially in young and nulliparous women.
**(b) False** The unfertilized ovum is autolysed in the fallopian tube some days prior to menstruation.
**(c) True** There is a wide variation, and a woman may find the loss excessive if it is an increase for her, even within this range.
**(d) False** Fifty years is the median age of the menopause.
**(e) False** Fluid retention precedes menstruation.

G 1

**4 (a) False** Ovulation occurs about 32 h after the onset of the LH surge (12 h after the peak).
**(b) True** The length of the luteal phase is fairly constant, whilst the follicular phase may vary considerably.
**(c) False** Progesterone secretion increases very shortly before ovulation, reaching its peak in the mid-luteal phase.
**(d) False** In some animals coitus stimulates ovulation, but not in the human.
**(e) True** Pseudocyesis is a spectacular example, but other emotional phenomena may prevent ovulation.

G 1

**5 (a) True** This may give rise to vaginitis.
**(b) False** There is an increase in FSH and LH production due to the loss of the oestrogen 'negative feedback'.
**(c) True** It is essential to exclude carcinoma of the endometrium.
**(d) True** Atrophic vaginitis is a common cause of dryness and discomfort which can be relieved with oestrogen either locally or systemically.
**(e) True**

G 1

6 Follicle-stimulating hormone (FSH):
   (a)  Is responsible for oestradiol production from the granulosa cells
   (b)  Brings about follicular rupture
   (c)  Is raised in polycystic ovary syndrome
   (d)  Is necessary for the initial stages of follicle development
   (e)  Is necessary for maintenance of the corpus luteum

7 The occlusive diaphragm:
   (a)  Should never be used for contraceptive purposes without contraceptive cream or jelly
   (b)  Has a similar Pearl index to the intra-uterine device
   (c)  Should be left *in situ* for at least 6 h after intercourse
   (d)  Is less reliable than the cervical (Dumas) cap
   (e)  May be particularly beneficial for prostitutes

8 The combined oral contraceptive:
   (a)  Predisposes to pelvic inflammatory disease
   (b)  Predisposes to benign breast and ovarian cysts
   (c)  Contains 0.2–0.5 mg of ethinyl oestradiol
   (d)  May be less effective in patients with epilepsy
   (e)  Works by causing an elevation in output of FSH and LH

9 Intra-uterine contraceptive devices:
   (a)  Should not be inserted at the time of suction termination of pregnancy
   (b)  Are radio-opaque
   (c)  Should be removed in early pregnancy if the threads are visible
   (d)  Should preferably be inserted at mid-cycle
   (e)  Are contra-indicated in patients with rheumatic heart disease

10 The following are absolute contra-indications to use of the combined oral contraceptive:
   (a)  Varicose veins
   (b)  A previous history of viral hepatitis
   (c)  A prosthetic heart valve
   (d)  Diabetes mellitus
   (e)  Carcinoma *in situ* of the cervix

**6 (a) True** The ovarian follicle is stimulated by FSH to produce oestradiol from the granulosa cells.

**(b) False** It is LH, released mid-cycle, which brings about the changes leading to oocyte release.

**(c) False** LH is raised in this condition, relative to the FSH level.

**(d) False** The very early stages of follicle development are hormone independent.

**(e) False** LH induces the change to promote corpus luteum formation, HCG stimulates its continuation.

G 1

**7 (a) True** The diaphragm by itself has little contraceptive effect and its function is to maintain a high concentration of spermicide at the cervical entrance.

**(b) False** It is less reliable than the intra-uterine device, having a Pearl index of 8–20, compared to less than 3 for the IUCD.

**(c) True** If intercourse is to take place repeatedly within this time it should be left for 6 h after the last intercourse.

**(d) False** The failure rates are much the same.

**(e) True** It protects against ascending infection and possibly to some extent against intra-epithelial neoplasia of the cervix, albeit less effectively than the condom.

G 11

**8 (a) False** It may be protective.

**(b) False** It protects against these conditions.

**(c) False** It contains 20–50 µg, i.e. 0.02–0.05 mg.

**(d) True** Hydantoins and barbiturates potentiate hepatic conjugation and excretion.

**(e) False** It has multiple modes of action but FSH and LH are suppressed.

G11

**9 (a) False** There is no apparent increased morbidity with this practice.

**(b) True** It may be helpful to locate an IUCD on X-ray, although ultrasound is more usually used to locate a 'missing' IUCD.

**(c) True** The risk of an IUCD causing miscarriage is greater if it is left *in situ*.

**(d) False** Shortly after menstruation is the recommended time.

**(e) True** Insertion predisposes to bacterial endocarditis.

G 11

**10 (a) False** Thrombo-embolism is not more likely unless the veins themselves are part of the post-thrombotic leg.

**(b) False** Provided liver function has returned to normal it is quite safe to prescribe oral contraceptives.

**(c) True** The added risk of thrombosis precludes the use of the oral contraceptive.

**(d) False** Insulin requirements may increase slightly but this is not an absolute contra-indication.

**(e) False** The oral contraceptive is not carcinogenic with regard to the cervix.

11 The following conditions are aggravated by the combined oral contraceptive:
   (a) Hirsuties
   (b) Endometriosis
   (c) Dysmenorrhoea
   (d) Premenstrual tension
   (e) Cervical erosion

12 The risks of the intra-uterine device in nulliparous women include:
   (a) Sterility
   (b) Elevated serum copper levels
   (c) Endometrial cancer
   (d) Ectopic pregnancy
   (e) Dyspareunia

13 Depo-provera:
   (a) Is usually used when contraception is required for more than two years
   (b) Causes amenorrhoea in more than 50% of cases
   (c) Does not prevent conception after 4 months
   (d) Should be given every 3 months
   (e) Prevents endometrial hyperplasia

14 Laparoscopic clip sterilization:
   (a) Can be reversed with greater success than vasectomy
   (b) May be surgically reversed with better results than surgery for
       postinfective tubal occlusion
   (c) Is associated with a failure rate of 1–2 in 1000
   (d) Has a higher failure rate when carried out at the time of termination of
       pregnancy
   (e) Always requires general anaesthesia.

**11 (a) False** Suppression of gonadotrophins diminishes ovarian androgen production and this, together with the direct effect of oestrogen may, if anything, cause a slight and gradual improvement in hirsuties.

**(b) False** Oestrogens by themselves aggravate endometriosis but the combined pill causes shrinkage of normal and ectopic endometrium.

**(c) False**
**(d) False** } Elimination of ovulation usually improves these symptoms.

**(e) True** Cervical erosion or ectropion commonly occurs in women who have been on the pill for some time.

G 11

**12 (a) True** Because of ascending infection giving rise to salpingitis, which may be silent.

**(b) False** The amount of copper ions released is minute and does not affect serum levels.

**(c) False** Although endometritis and increased menstrual loss may occur, there is no evidence to suggest endometrial cancer is a risk.

**(d) True** The risk is greater than with barrier methods or ovulation inhibitors. The risk per cycle is not increased in comparison with women using no contraception, but the cumulative risk is greater.

**(e) True** Dyspareunia probably occurs in relation to mild infection.

G 11

**13 (a) False** It is licensed for short-term use only (although many authorities consider it safe for longer term use).

**(b) True** Its effectiveness for at least 3 months nicely covers the risk period of rubella vaccination to an unplanned pregnancy.

**(c) False** Duration of action is variable after 3 months.

**(d) True** Although the duration of action may be as long as 6 months, 3 months is the maximal period on which one can rely.

**(e) True** Like other progestogens, it suppresses endometrium.

G 11

**14 (a) True** Antisperm antibodies reduce the success of vasectomy reversal.

**(b) True** Eighty per cent patency and 50% pregnancy rates can be expected after microscopic re-anastomosis and even better results have been reported from selected centres. The outlook for surgical repair after tubal diathermy is very poor.

**(c) True** Couples should be warned of this.

**(d) True** The increased vascularity if the woman is or has recently been pregnant increases the risk of re-canalization.

**(e) False** Local anaesthesia can be used.

G 11 & 14

**15** The following structures are correct:

(a)

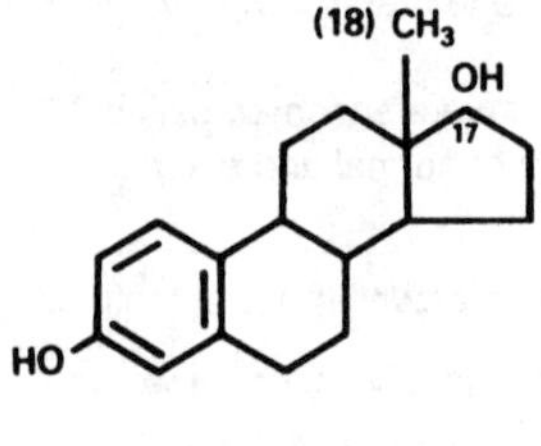

Oestrone

(b)

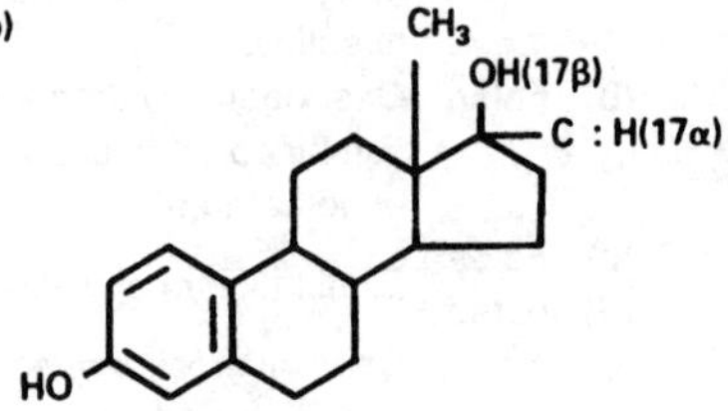

17α-Ethinyloestradiol

(c)

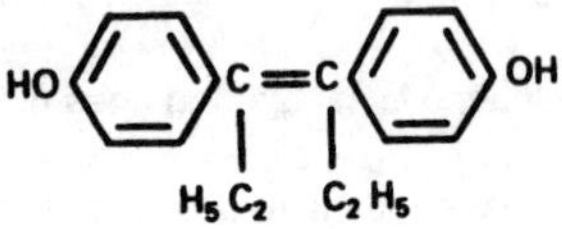

Diethylstilboestrol

(d)

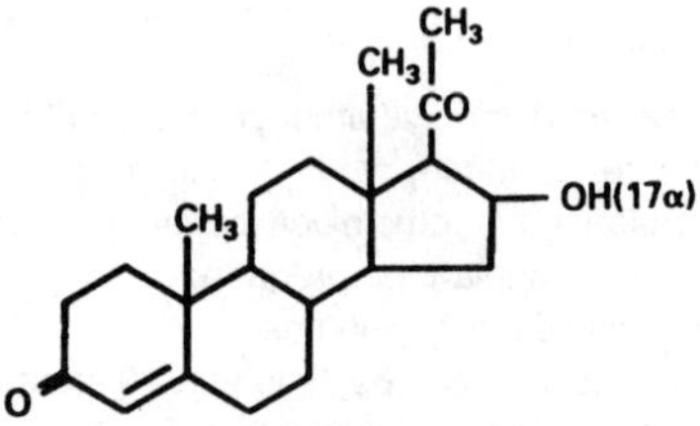

17α-Hydroxyprogesterone

(e)

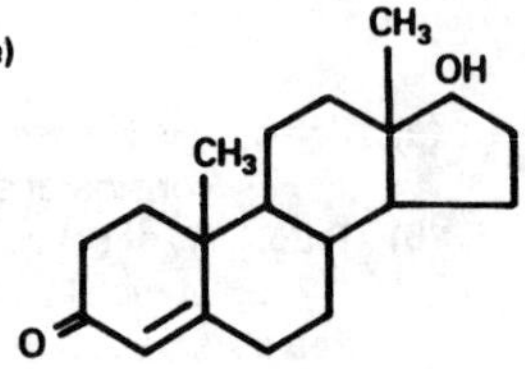

Testosterone

**16** Bromocriptine:
  (a) Is an analogue of prolactin
  (b) Is used to treat hyperprolactinaemia
  (c) Is a potent cause of multiple pregnancy
  (d) May cause hypotension
  (e) Effectively inhibits lactation after delivery

**17** The following hormones are active when given by mouth:
  (a) Oestradiol benzoate
  (b) Equine conjugated oestrogens
  (c) Ethinyloestradiol
  (d) Norethisterone
  (e) 17-Hydroxyprogesterone

15 **(a) False** This is oestradiol.
   **(b) True**
   **(c) True**
   **(d) False** The hydroxyl group should be in position 17, not 16 as shown here.
   **(e) True**

16 **(a) False** It is a derivative of ergot alkaloid.
   **(b) True** It has an inhibitory effect on pituitary cells and so less prolactin is produced.
   **(c) False** It is not associated with multiple ovulation.
   **(d) True** This is less likely to occur if the dosage is increased slowly, and the tablet given at night.
   **(e) True** Rebound lactation may however occur if it is stopped abruptly.
   
   **G 13**

17 **(a) False** Oestradiol valerate is orally active, and benzoate is used as an injectable preparation.
   **(b) True** This is a mixture of oestrone, oestradiol and oestriol, most of which is converted to oestradiol.
   **(c) True** The addition of an ethinyl group to the $17\alpha$ position results in a very potent orally active oestrogen.
   **(d) True** This is a very active derivative of nortestosterone.
   **(e) False** This is only active when given by intramuscular injection.   **G 13**

18 Therapeutic indications for progestogens include:
   (a) Endometriosis
   (b) Fibroids
   (c) Endometrial carcinoma
   (d) Habitual abortion
   (e) Dysfunctional uterine bleeding

19 Gonadotrophin-releasing hormone (GnRH):
   (a) Stimulates release of FSH as well as LH
   (b) Is a peptide of high molecular weight
   (c) May be administered by single injection to stimulate ovulation
   (d) When given in high dosage causes pituitary desensitization and a fall in FSH and LH
   (e) Is produced by acidophilic cells of the anterior pituitary

20 The following are indications for oestrogen treatment:
   (a) Fibroids
   (b) Atrophic vulval dystrophy
   (c) Postmenopausal vaginitis
   (d) Threatened abortion
   (e) Ovarian dysgenesis

21 The following hormones are predominantly oestrogens:
   (a) Dienoestrol
   (b) Norethynodrel
   (c) Premarin
   (d) Androstenedione
   (e) Norgestrel

22 The following values of a semen analysis indicate *abnormal* semen quality:
   (a) Volume of less than 2 ml
   (b) Density of 40 million/ml
   (c) Motility of 40%
   (d) Abnormal forms of 40%
   (e) Liquefaction complete in 30 min

**18 (a) True** Continuous administration suppresses cyclical bleeding from the endometrium, both normal and ectopic.

**(b) False** Fibroids may enlarge if progestogens are given.

**(c) True** Regression of metastases (and the primary tumour) occurs in at least a proportion of cases.

**(d) False** Although injections of progesterone have been widely used in the past for this purpose, there is no evidence of their efficacy.

**(e) True** It is particularly effective in cystic glandular hyperplasia.

**G 13**

**19 (a) True** It is secreted in a pulsatile fashion and stimulates release of FSH and LH.

**(b) False** It is a low molecular weight decapeptide.

**(c) False** Its activity depends on pulsatility, both physiologically and when used therapeutically. Continuous administration diminishes gondatotrophin secretion by down regulating its own receptor.

**(d) True** This blocking action is utilized with the synthetic GnRH analogues to render women amenorrhoeic.

**(e) False** It is produced by neurosecretory cells in the hypothalamus.

**G 13**

**20 (a) False** Indeed, oestrogens may accelerate the growth of fibroids.

**(b) False** Although this condition appears after the menopause, it does not respond to oestrogen treatment. Hydrocortisone and testosterone creams are used for symptomatic cases.

**(c) True** Oestrogen is effective either orally or vaginally.

**(d) False** The use of synthetic oestrogens in pregnancy predisposes the exposed female fetus to cervical and vaginal neoplasia in later life.

**(e) True** Oestrogen will promote development of breasts and secondary sexual characteristics in these patients.

**G 13**

**21 (a) True** This is synthetic oestrogen, active orally, but often used for local vaginal action.

**(b) False** This is a synthetic progestogen.

**(c) True** This is conjugated equine oestrogen.

**(d) False** This is a weak androgen.

**(e) False** This is a progestogen.

**G 13**

**22 (a) True** The normal volume is 2–5 ml.

**(b) False** The count is below 20 million to justify diagnosing oligospermia.

**(c) True** Motility should be at least 50%.

**(d) False** More than 70% of sperm need to be abnormal forms to indicate likely subfertility on account of morphology.

**(e) False** This is the normal liquefaction time.

**G 11**

23 Gonadotrophin-releasing hormone (GnRH) agonists:
   (a) Must be given by pump
   (b) Cause initial gonadotrophin release
   (c) Are effective in treatment of endometriosis
   (d) Cause bone loss
   (e) Relieve menopausal hot flushes

24 The following are acceptable methods for confirmation of ovulation:
   (a) Basal body temperature drop at least 0.5°C on the 14th day
   (b) A day-21 blood progesterone level
   (c) Histological examination of premenstrual endometrial biopsy
   (d) Blood oestrogen level on the 13th day
   (e) Demonstration of spinnbarkheit in cervical mucus

25 Tubal patency may properly be demonstrated by:
   (a) Hysterosalpingography
   (b) Air insufflation
   (c) Laparoscopy and methylene-blue dye insufflation
   (d) Computerized tomography (CT) scan
   (e) Hysteroscopy

26 The following are recognized complications of treatment of anovulatory infertility:
   (a) Multiple pregnancy
   (b) Ectopic pregnancy
   (c) Cervical mucus hostility
   (d) Postural hypotension
   (e) Ascites

27 Clomiphene citrate:
   (a) Results in decreased cervical mucus production
   (b) Blocks FSH release
   (c) Results in increased GnRH release
   (d) Directly stimulates follicular growth
   (e) May result in ovarian hyperstimulation

23 (a) **False** GnRH itself is given by pump. The analogue (agonist) is given by nasal spray or injection.

(b) **True** They are *agonists*. Commercially available antagonists are under development.

(c) **True** With continued use they 'down-regulate' the pituitary. Endometriosis will usually recur when treatment is stopped.

(d) **True** Due to hypoestrogenism.

(e) **False** Flushes are a side-effect.

**G 13**

24 (a) **False** A rise in temperature of $0.5°C$ must be seen to be maintained over the last 14 days of the cycle.

(b) **True** Progesterone reaches a mid-luteal peak which is maintained until just before menstruation.

(c) **True** Secretory changes in the endometrium only occur after ovulation.

(d) **False** Oestrogen levels indicate follicular development, but not ovulation.

(e) **False** This is a pre-ovulatory phenomenon dependent on oestrogen.

**G 11**

25 (a) **True** Injection of a radio-opaque dye is usually screened on an image intensifier prior to taking X-ray pictures.

(b) **False** Insufflation with $CO_2$ is acceptable, but with air there is a grave danger of air embolus.

(c) **True** In many centres this is now the method of choice for assessing tubal patency.

(d) **False** CT is not helpful for this procedure.

(e) **False** Hysteroscopy examines the uterine cavity, not the tubes.

**G 11**

26 (a) **True** Both clomiphene and gonadotrophin therapy may cause multiple ovulation and hence multiple pregnancy.

(b) **False** Tubal surgery and *in vitro* fertilization may result in ectopic pregnancy but not ovulatory stimulation *per se*.

(c) **True** Clomiphene, because of its anti-oestrogenic effect, may render cervical mucous hostile.

(d) **True** This is a classical side-effect when bromocriptine treatment is started.

(e) **True** Hyperstimulation with gonadotrophin may lead to ovarian cyst formation with ascites.

**G 11**

27 (a) **True** The anti-oestrogenic effect of clomiphene may render cervical mucus thick.

(b) **False** It is an anti-oestrogen which increases gonadotrophic production.

(c) **True** It blocks the oestrogen receptor sites in the hypothalamus, and so stimulates increasing GnRH release.

(d) **False** Its actions are mediated by restoration of FSH secretion.

(e) **True** The full-blown clinical syndrome is very rare with clomiphene used by itself.

**G 11**

28 In male factor infertility:
  (a) Men with hypogonadotrophic hypogonadism respond to mesterolone (testosterone analogue)
  (b) Tamoxifen may increase spermatogenesis
  (c) Steroids may decrease antisperm antibody levels
  (d) The postcoital test is usually positive
  (e) May be helped by ICSI


29 During a vaginal examination, the diagnosis of vaginismus is suggested by:
  (a) Profuse vaginal discharge
  (b) Involuntary spasm of levator ani muscles
  (c) Involuntary abduction of the hips
  (d) Congenital vaginal stenosis
  (e) Imperforate hymen


30 Orgasmic dysfunction in women can be due to:
  (a) Neurological problems
  (b) Vaginismus
  (c) Inadequate clitoral stimulation
  (d) Fear of losing control
  (e) Pregnancy


31 Termination of pregnancy:
  (a) May legally be performed at any gestation when there are severe fetal abnormalities
  (b) Can be performed using prostaglandins
  (c) Must be approved by three independent medical practitioners
  (d) May be carried out using Mifepristone (RU 486) up to 12 weeks gestation
  (e) Is safely carried out by suction before 14 weeks gestation


32 In threatened abortion:
  (a) The uterine size is typically less than expected for the period of gestation
  (b) Progesterone therapy is useful
  (c) Pain is absent
  (d) Vaginal bleeding is present in most cases
  (e) Bed rest may prevent miscarriage

28 **(a) False**   Gonadotrophins are necessary.
    **(b) True**   But the fertility rate is not improved.
    **(c) True**   An increase in fertility is also reported, but relatively high dosage of steroids is required.
    **(d) False**   A negative postcoital test is quite often the first pointer to male factor infertility.
    **(e) True**   Intracytoplasmic injection allows fertilization of oocytes with remarkably low sperm densities.

**G 11**

29 **(a) False**   Vaginismus is an involuntary spasm of the levator ani due to fear. Vaginitis, although uncomfortable, does not lead to spasm.
    **(b) True**   It is usually fear of pain that causes the spasm.
    **(c) False**   It is the adduction of the hips that prevents examination.
    **(d) False**   Mechanical vaginal obstruction does not cause the 'withdrawal
    **(e) False**   response' of vaginismus.

**G 11**

30 **(a) True**   Long-standing diabetes and multiple sclerosis are recognized causes of sexual disorders.
    **(b) False**   Women with vaginismus are usually orgasmic with clitoral stimulation.
    **(c) True**   These are the common causes of anorgasmia.
    **(d) True**
    **(e) False**   Some women may fear that orgasm will be harmful to the pregnancy, but there is no evidence to that effect.

**G 11**

31 **(a) True**   The 1992 changes to the abortion law allow termination for fetal abnormalities at any gestation, but restrict termination for other indications to below 24 weeks.
    **(b) True**   Prostaglandins, either by pessary or extra-amniotic injection, are used to induce mid-trimester abortion.
    **(c) False**   Two practitioners must certify that there are legal grounds for termination.
    **(d) False**   Mifepristone must be used in conjunction with a prostaglandin, and is only licensed for use prior to 9 weeks gestation.
    **(e) True**   This is the most widely used method for first trimester termination.

**G 10**

32 **(a) False**   This is a feature of missed abortion.
    **(b) False**   Progesterone has been shown not to help and may interfere with external genital development in continuing pregnancies.
    **(c) True**   By definition, a threatened abortion is bleeding in early pregnancy without pain.
    **(d) False**   Vaginal bleeding is *always* present, by definition.
    **(e) False**   Bed rest has been shown to confer no benefit.

**G 10**

33 Causes of first trimester abortion include:
 (a) Malaria infection
 (b) Rubella
 (c) Syphilis
 (d) XO karyotype in the embryo
 (e) Trisomy 21 in the embryo

34 Septic abortion:
 (a) May result from exposure to gonorrhoea during pregnancy
 (b) Is frequently due to a combination of coliforms and bacteroides
 (c) Is more likely to lead to septic shock than salpingitis or pelvic abscess in a non-pregnant patient
 (d) Should be treated by immediate curettage of the uterus in all cases
 (e) Is a less common cause of maternal death in Britain than it was 20 years ago

35 In the diagnosis of ectopic pregnancy:
 (a) A ruptured corpus luteum cyst may cause identical clinical features
 (b) Vaginal bleeding will be present in 99% of all cases
 (c) The standard pregnancy test is very useful
 (d) Pain usually precedes vaginal bleeding
 (e) A history of 10 weeks amenorrhoea and pain in a patient who usually has 28-day cycles is highly suggestive

36 Ectopic pregnancy:
 (a) Is associated with uterine enlargement
 (b) Is situated in the ovary in about 0.5% of all cases
 (c) Is more dangerous when it is situated in the isthmus of the fallopian tube
 (d) Can only be diagnosed after it has ruptured
 (e) Is a complication of assisted conception

**33 (a) True** Any high fever can cause abortion but malaria is particularly likely to do so because plasmodium parasitizes the chorio-decidual space.

**(b) True** Although the association between rubella and congenital defects is better known, acute rubella may result in miscarriage.

**(c) False** The spirochaete does not cross the placenta until after 20 weeks of pregnancy.

**(d) True** This is the commonest chromosomal abnormality in abortion material.

**(e) True** Eighty per cent of 'Down's' embryos are aborted.    **G 10**

**34 (a) False** The cervical plug is a very effective barrier to ascending infection during pregnancy.

**(b) True** Since these organisms are commonly present in the vagina and perineum, they often infect an incomplete abortion.

**(c) True** Pregnant patients are particularly predisposed to endotoxic shock.

**(d) False** (i) Where bleeding is not heavy and the patient has a very high temperature, curettage should be deferred for 6–12 h to give time for antibiotics to take effect. Immediate surgical interference may lead to septic shock. Any pieces of infective material in the cervix should, however, be removed with sponge forceps.
(ii) If the uterus is over 14 weeks in size, contractions should be induced by an oxytocin infusion.

**(e) True** This is due, at least in part, to the introduction of legal abortion.
    **G 10**

**35 (a) True** This causes intraperitoneal haemorrhage (which is often considerable) after a short period of amenorrhoea. The differential diagnosis is difficult, and may only be clarified by laparoscopy.

**(b) False** It is present in about 85% of cases. It is often absent in those acute ectopics with intraperitoneal rupture of the isthmus.

**(c) False** It is only positive in 50% of cases; the more sensitive βHCG test may be useful.

**(d) True** Pain usually comes first, in contrast with spontaneous abortion.

**(e) False** Patients with ectopic pregnancy usually have a short history of amenorrhoea – 6–8 weeks from the start of the last period. Ten weeks would suggest inevitable abortion.
    **G 10**

**36 (a) True** Although uterine enlargement occurs under the influence of oestrogen and progesterone, it is not as large as an intra-uterine pregnancy.

**(b) True** Ovarian implantation is a rare site for ectopic pregnancy.

**(c) True** This tends to lead to tubal rupture and massive intraperitoneal haemorrhage. Ampullary implantation more often leads to 'tubal abortion' with a more gradual accumulation of blood.

**(d) False** The increasing use of sensitive βHCG tests and transvaginal ultrasound often allows diagnosis of ectopic pregnancy prior to rupture.

**(e) True** There is a three-fold increased incidence with IVF and GIFT.
    **G 10**

37 Cervical incompetence:
   (a) Typically causes painful abortions
   (b) Typically causes mid-trimester abortion
   (c) Is treated by cervical cerclage which is best performed early in the second trimester
   (d) May be caused by hydramnios
   (e) May lead to premature rupture of the membranes

38 Mid-trimester abortion with prostaglandins:
   (a) Is illegal after 20 weeks gestation
   (b) May result in uterine rupture
   (c) May cause cervical laceration
   (d) May cause convulsions
   (e) Usually takes more than 24 h

39 In the UK termination of pregnancy requires:
   (a) Consent from the partner as well as the woman
   (b) A surgical operation
   (c) Consent from guardian of a minor
   (d) Agreement of any two doctors
   (e) Notification of the Department of Health

40 Pregnancy may be terminated using:
   (a) Prostaglandin inhibitors
   (b) Progesterone inhibitors
   (c) Suction evacuation
   (d) Laminaria tents
   (e) Beta-blocking agents

41 In Turner's syndrome:
   (a) A chromosomal structure of 45 XY is characteristic
   (b) Secondary amenorrhoea is usual
   (c) Coarctation of the aorta may occur
   (d) The ovaries are multicystic
   (e) Pubic hair is absent

37 **(a)** **False** The 'incompetent' cervix dilates easily; thus abortion is relatively pain-free in typical cases.

   **(b)** **True** It is doubtful if it is ever a cause of first trimester loss.

   **(c)** **True** First trimester abortion for other reasons is common (15–20% of all pregnancies); thus cerclage is best delayed until the second trimester.

   **(d)** **False** Hydramnios, however, leads to premature delivery in its own right.

   **(e)** **True** The incompetent cervix typically presents with painless dilatation, followed by rupture of the membranes.

**G 10**

38 **(a)** **False** Twenty-four weeks is the upper limit of gestation, and for gross fetal abnormality, the pregnancy may be terminated at any stage.

   **(b)** **False** The uterus does not rupture with termination.

   **(c)** **True** Unduly strong contractions may cause cervical laceration.

   **(d)** **False** Excessive use of oxytocin may cause water intoxication and convulsions, but not with the use of prostaglandins alone.

   **(e)** **False** Abortion is usually complete within 12–24 h.

**G 10**

39 **(a)** **False** Only the woman's consent is required.

   **(b)** **False** Prostaglandins and anti-progesterones are but two of the pharmaceutical agents which may be used for termination.

   **(c)** **True** If the girl is under 16 years, the parents must be consulted, even if the patient objects.

   **(d)** **False** Only *registered* medical practitioners who are not in partnership may sign the certificate (except in an emergency procedure when only one signature is required).

   **(e)** **True** The doctor terminating the pregnancy has an obligation to fill in the prescribed notification form and send it to the Department of Health.

**G 10**

40 **(a)** **False** It is prostaglandins themselves which may be used.

   **(b)** **True** Mifepristone, an anti-progesterone, may be used in conjunction with prostaglandin.

   **(c)** **True** This method can be used up to 13–14 weeks, or even later by a skilled operator.

   **(d)** **True** Although not often used nowadays, these may have a place when the cervix is difficult to dilate.

   **(e)** **False** These relax uterine contractions in later pregnancy.

**G 10**

41 **(a)** **False** 45 XO is the commonest karyotype. Mosaics such as XO, XX may also occur.

   **(b)** **False** There is primary amenorrhoea.

   **(c)** **True** It is well recognized to occur in association with Turner's syndrome.

   **(d)** **False** The ovaries are streak-like structures.

   **(e)** **True** There is a lack of all secondary sexual characteristics.

**G 3**

42 Patients with the following conditions typically present with primary amenorrhoea:
  (a) Uterus didelphys
  (b) Imperforate hymen
  (c) Anorexia nervosa
  (d) Testicular feminization
  (e) Untreated congenital adrenal hyperplasia

43 The following investigations may be relevant in cases of amenorrhoea:
  (a) Skull X-ray
  (b) Pregnancy test
  (c) Thyroid function tests
  (d) Glucose tolerance test
  (e) GnRH estimation

44 In the polycystic ovary syndrome:
  (a) Obesity is common
  (b) There is loss of body hair
  (c) LH levels are low
  (d) Irregular widely spaced menstruation is typical
  (e) Clomiphene may restore ovulation and menstruation

45 In testicular feminization:
  (a) The chromosome status is XXY
  (b) The gonads should be removed after puberty
  (c) The patient adopts a male role and appearance
  (d) Breasts are absent
  (e) The voice is female

46 Postcoital bleeding may be a sign of:
  (a) Fibroids
  (b) Adenomatous polyps
  (c) Cervical erosion
  (d) Dysplasia of the cervix
  (e) Carcinoma in situ

47 Heavy, but regular, periods are a likely feature of:
  (a) Fibroids
  (b) Carcinoma of the cervix
  (c) Dysfunctional uterine bleeding
  (d) Myxoedema
  (e) Hypertension

**42 (a) False** There is no effect on menstruation.
**(b) True** Strictly speaking this causes cryptomenorrhoea (i.e. retention of menstrual secretion) but it is a differential diagnosis of primary amenorrhoea.
**(c) False** This causes secondary amenorrhoea.
**(d) True** The uterus is absent.
**(e) True** Once treated with corticosteroids, normal menstruation occurs.

**G 3**

**43 (a) True** This is often done to visualize the pituitary fossa.
**(b) True** One must never overlook the possibility of pregnancy.
**(c) True** Both myxoedema and hyperthyroidism may cause amenorrhoea.
**(d) False** Although severe diabetes may cause amenorrhoea, it is unlikely to be a presenting symptom.
**(e) False** GnRH stimulation tests are sometimes carried out, but GnRH assay is not routinely available.

**G 8**

**44 (a) True** When the condition was first described by Stein and Leventhal, obesity was thought to be invariably present. It is now recognized that not all women with PCO are obese.
**(b) False** There is usually hirsuties.
**(c) False** There is a relatively high LH level compared with FSH.
**(d) True** In the most extreme forms, there is complete amenorrhoea, but oligomenorrhoea would be the most frequent pattern.
**(e) True** Clomiphene induces ovulation in about 70% of women with PCO.

**G 11**

**45 (a) False** Chromosome karyotype is XY.
**(b) True** There is a 5% risk of development of dysgerminoma.
**(c) False** They are invariably female in appearance.
**(d) False** The breasts are fairly well developed after puberty.
**(e) True** There is androgen insensitivity and so no masculination of the larynx takes place.

**G 3**

**46 (a) True** From a fibroid polyp.
**(b) True** A benign endometrial polyp may, rarely, extrude through the cervix.
**(c) True** The columnar epithelium of an erosion is more likely to bleed slightly than squamous epithelium.
**(d) False** The naked eye appearance of cervical dysplasia and carcinoma *in*
**(e) False** *situ* is normal, and they do not cause symptoms.

**G 5**

**47 (a) True** They are a very common cause of menorrhagia.
**(b) False** This usually causes irregular bleeding.
**(c) True** The ovulatory forms of dysfunctional uterine bleeding are often regular. Anovulatory dysfunctional bleeding seen with severe polycystic ovary syndrome and at the extremes of reproductive life is irregular.
**(d) True** In more severe cases of myxoedema, amenorrhoea may occur.
**(e) False** Hypertension is not a cause of heavy periods.

**G 8**

48 Cystic glandular hyperplasia:
  (a)  Is associated with low oestrogen levels
  (b)  May predispose to endometrial carcinoma
  (c)  Is caused by a virus transmitted in cheese
  (d)  Occurs with ovulatory failure
  (e)  Generally occurs postmenopausally

49 Premenstrual tension syndrome:
  (a)  Mostly occurs in women under 25 years
  (b)  Is often accompanied by depression and irritability
  (c)  Is only relieved when the menstrual flow is completed
  (d)  Is exacerbated by psychosocial factors
  (e)  May be associated with acts of crime

50 Effective treatments for primary (spasmodic) dysmenorrhoea include:
  (a)  Diuretics
  (b)  Flufenamic acid
  (c)  Flenfluramine
  (d)  Combined contraceptive pills
  (e)  Presacral neurectomy

51 Candida infection has a recognized association with:
  (a)  Oral contraception
  (b)  Chronic renal disease
  (c)  Antibiotic treatment
  (d)  The menopause
  (e)  Cervical dysplasia

48  (a)  **False**  In the early phase of the menopause, oestrogen levels are maintained, but ovulation does not occur. This leads to a thickened cystic endometrium which sheds irregularly. Lack of progesterone means that the normal tortuosity and constrictor effect on spiral arterioles is lost.

    (b)  **True**  The endometrial hyperplasia may be atypical with danger of progression to carcinoma.

    (c)  **False**  The histological appearance is sometimes described as being like 'Swiss cheese'. There the connection ends!

    (d)  **True**  The lack of ovulation and absence of progesterone leads to a prolonged high level of oestrogen.

    (e)  **False**  It occurs in puberty and peri-menopausally.

**G 8**

49  (a)  **False**  It is commoner in women over 30 years.

    (b)  **True**  The cause of the emotional disturbance is not known.

    (c)  **False**  It is usually relieved by the *start* of the menstrual flow.

    (d)  **True**  In the management of the condition, recognition of adverse contributory factors is important.

    (e)  **True**  There is an increased incidence of shoplifting, etc., and even major acts of violence are said to occur more often in the premenstrual phase.

**G 8**

50  (a)  **False**  Diuretics may be helpful in cyclical oedema, but not dysmenorrhoea.

    (b)  **True**  Prostaglandin inhibitors such as this may diminish uterine contractions and be helpful.

    (c)  **False**  This agent is an appetite suppressant.

    (d)  **True**  Suppression of ovulation nearly always relieves dysmenorrhoea.

    (e)  **True**  This operation is not often performed now, as simpler treatments are usually effective.

**G 8**

51  (a)  **True**  The oral contraceptive pill probably induces subtle changes in vaginal flora or pH which increases susceptibility to Candida infection.

    (b)  **False**

    (c)  **True**  This commonly precedes Candida infection, because it alters vaginal flora.

    (d)  **False**  Loss of glycogen in vaginal epithelium occurs at the menopause, and vaginal Candida infection becomes less likely.

    (e)  **False**  This is in contrast to the typical sexually transmitted infections such as trichomonas and papilloma virus.

**G 5**

52 The following organisms are known causes of pelvic inflammatory disease:
  (a) *Streptococcus pyogenes*
  (b) Herpes simplex
  (c) Chlamydia
  (d) *Clostridium welchii*
  (e) Trichomonas

53 Tuberculosis of the female genital tract:
  (a) Most commonly affects the fallopian tubes
  (b) Is usually sexually transmitted
  (c) May cause ascites
  (d) Causes infertility
  (e) Is best diagnosed by taking an endometrial biopsy in the first half of the cycle

54 In women with syphilis:
  (a) The incubation may be as long as 3 months
  (b) A chancre will be seen in most cases
  (c) If the VDRL (venereal disease research laboratory slide test) is positive, the TPHA will be negative
  (d) General paralysis of the insane may result
  (e) Tetracyclines may be used for treatment

55 Chlamydial infection is:
  (a) The most common cause of sexually transmitted diseases (STD)
  (b) Caused by an intracellular organism
  (c) Silent in over half of cases
  (d) Sensitive to metronidazole
  (e) A possible cause of pneumonia in infants

56 Human immunodeficiency virus (HIV) carriers:
  (a) Are always serum antibody positive
  (b) Have a better prognosis with treatment
  (c) Cannot transmit the disease until they develop the clinical syndrome
  (d) Transmit the virus to the fetus in over 80% of cases
  (e) Will almost certainly not develop the disease

57 Gonorrhoea:
  (a) Infects the vaginal epithelium
  (b) May cause arthritis
  (c) May be symptomless
  (d) Is diagnosed by a serological test
  (e) Crosses the placenta

52 (a) **True**   The organism is often responsible for postabortion or postdelivery infection.
(b) **False**   Herpes simplex infection is confined to the vagina and cervix.
(c) **True**   This and *Neiserria gonococci* cause more than two-thirds of cases, but super-infection with other organisms usually occurs.
(d) **True**   May occur following criminal abortion.
(e) **False**   Affects the vagina only.

**G 5**

53 (a) **True**   The tubes and endometrium are invariably affected.
(b) **False**   It is nearly always secondary to pulmonary tuberculosis.
(c) **True**   This is now a rare cause of ascites in the UK.
(d) **True**   The tubes are almost invariably infected and even after full chemotherapy, restoration of fertility is unusual.
(e) **False**   It is necessary to take a biopsy in the second half of the cycle when the granulomata have had time to develop.

**G5**

54 (a) **True**   The incubation period may be from 9 to 90 days.
(b) **False**   Women usually present with secondary disease because the chancre is not noticed as it is not exposed.
(c) **False**   The VDRL is based on IgM and becomes negative more rapidly after successful treatment.
(d) **True**   This is fortunately now a rare manifestation of neurosyphilis.
(e) **True**   This is second-line treatment, for those sensitive to penicillin.

**G 5**

55 (a) **True**   Infection due to Chlamydia is now the most common sexually transmitted disease.
(b) **True**   It is a Gram-negative intracellular obligate bacterium.
(c) **True**   It is commonly harboured in the cervix without symptoms.
(d) **False**   It is sensitive to tetracycline and erythromycin.
(e) **True**   The more common neonatal infection is ophthalmic neonatorum.

**G 5**

56 (a) **False**   Most cases develop antibodies within 3 months of infection.
(b) **True**   Many of the opportunistic infections may be prevented or improved with appropriate antibiotics, and anti-viral agents may slow the progression.
(c) **False**   An HIV-positive patient is just as potentially infective as someone with AIDS.
(d) **False**   Transplacental spread occurs in less than half of cases.
(e) **False**   At the present time, virtually all HIV-positive patients will eventually progress to AIDS.

**G 5**

57 (a) **False**   It infects glandular epithelium such as the cervix or urethra.
(b) **True**   Blood-borne spread to joints, endocardium and iris are all rare.
(c) **True**   In women symptoms are often mild or non-existent.
(d) **False**   The gonoccocal complement fixation test is notoriously unreliable and does not become positive until some weeks after infection.
(e) **False**   Gonoccocal ophthalmia may be acquired by the baby during delivery, but the organism does not cross the placenta.

**G 5**

58 Tubal damage is a recognized complication of:
   (a) Asymptomatic chlamydial salpingitis
   (b) Pneumococcal salpingitis
   (c) Intra-uterine devices
   (d) Ovarian cystectomy
   (e) Actinomycosis

59 Acceptable treatment for uterine fibroids includes:
   (a) No treatment
   (b) Myomechtomy during pregnancy if red degeneration occurs
   (c) Cyclical oestrogen treatment
   (d) Vaginal myomectomy
   (e) Caesarean hysterectomy

60 Fibroids:
   (a) May protrude through the cervix
   (b) Are composed mostly of fibrous tissue
   (c) Are more common in infertile patients
   (d) Are rare in Negroes
   (e) Commonly arise from the cervix

61 Complications of fibroids include:
   (a) Intraperitoneal haemorrhage
   (b) Endometrial carcinoma
   (c) Obstructed labour
   (d) Polycythaemia
   (e) Recurrent abortion

62 Endometriosis is a recognized cause of:
   (a) Deep dyspareunia
   (b) Amenorrhoea
   (c) Dysmenorrhoea
   (d) Postmenopausal bleeding
   (e) Painful laparotomy scar

63 Endometriosis:
   (a) Is the commonest cause of chronic lower abdominal pain in young women
   (b) Most frequently involves the ovaries
   (c) Often flares up during pregnancy
   (d) Is associated with subfertility
   (e) Is more common in Negro races

**58 (a) True**    Ascending infection can occur, resulting in tubal damage without any symptoms.

**(b) False**

**(c) True**    Ascending pelvic infections are more common especially in nulliparous women.

**(d) True**    The fimbriae may become involved in peritubal adhesions.

**(e) True**    This is a well-recognized infection in association with intra-uterine devices.

**G 5**

**59 (a) True**    If tumours are small (less than the size of a 12-week pregnancy) and asymptomatic, this is the appropriate management.

**(b) False**    This can be highly dangerous, causing severe haemorrhage, and is likely to initiate labour.

**(c) False**    This tends to cause enlargement of fibroids.

**(d) True**    This is appropriate for pedunculated submucous fibroids.

**(e) True**    If no further pregnancies are desired.

**G 6**

**60 (a) True**    Submucosal fibroids may become polypoid and be extruded through the cervix where they ulcerate and become infected.

**(b) False**    They are composed mostly of smooth muscle.

**(c) True**    They are more common in people who are subfertile and, once formed, they may contribute further to subfertility.

**(d) False**    They are three times more common than in Caucasians.

**(e) False**    Only 2% arise in this site.

**G 6**

**61 (a) True**    From rupture of a surface vessel.

**(b) False**    Sarcoma is found in 0.2%.

**(c) True**    A pelvic fibroid may obstruct labour.

**(d) True**    This is probably due to erythropoetin secretion by the tumour.

**(e) True**    Submucous fibroids, in particular, may interfere with implantation and cause abortion.

**G 6**

**62 (a) True**    This is one of the classical features along with dysmenorrhoea, pain and menorrhagia.

**(b) False**    Significant hormone imbalance is not a feature.

**(c) True**    Cyclical bleeding into or from the deposits causes pain prior to and during menstruation.

**(d) False**    Endometriotic deposits usually regress after the menopause.

**(e) True**    Rarely, ectopic endometrium may appear in scars.

**G 7**

**63 (a) False**    In most cases of chronic pelvic pain, no cause is found.

**(b) True**    The peritoneum of the broad ligament and pouch of Douglas is the second commonest site.

**(c) False**    The disease regresses during pregnancy.

**(d) True**    The mechanism by which it does so is not clearly understood as ovulation and tubal patency are usually maintained.

**(e) False**    Fibroids are more common in the Negro race; endometriosis in Caucasians.

**G 7**

64 The following are useful for the treatment of endometriosis:
   (a) Danazol
   (b) Dydrogesterone
   (c) GnRH analogues
   (d) The oral contraceptive
   (e) Prednisolone

65 Chronic pelvic pain:
   (a) May be a manifestation of underlying psychological distress
   (b) Should always be investigated by laparotomy
   (c) Is by definition cyclical
   (d) Is a frequent symptom of chronic pelvic inflammatory disease
   (e) Is most common in postmenopausal women

66 Low backache in women is associated with:
   (a) A retroverted uterus
   (b) Premenstrual syndrome
   (c) Gynaecological abnormalities more often than musculoskeletal problems
   (d) Long-standing endometriosis
   (e) Pregnancy

67 The following vulval conditions cause pruritus vulvae:
   (a) Hypertrophic dystrophy
   (b) Lymphogranuloma venereum
   (c) Condylomata acuminata
   (d) Syphilitic chancre
   (e) Threadworms

68 The vulva:
   (a) May be the site of primary trichomonas infection
   (b) Is the site of 5% of all malignant growths of the female reproductive tract
   (c) Becomes atrophic after the menopause
   (d) May be the site for lichen sclerosis et atrophicus
   (e) May be involved in primary, secondary and tertiary syphilis

64 (a) **True**   Danazol, a weak androgen with anti-oestrogenic action,
suppresses menstruation, but may have severe side-effects.

(b) **True**   This synthetic progestogen also suppresses menstruation if given
continuously. Side-effects include weight gain and fluid retention.

(c) **True**   These act by suppressing pituitary gonadotrophin production, and
amenorrhoea results.

(d) **True**   The beneficial effect is due to the progestogen.

(e) **False**   Corticosteroids have no effect on endometriosis.

G 7

65 (a) **True**   Psychogenic pain should not be diagnosed until organic
causes have been excluded.

(b) **False**   Ultrasound and laparoscopy are the two most useful
investigations.

(c) **False**   Dysmenorrhoea, mittelschmerz and pelvic congestion are
examples of cyclical pain, but other causes are often
non-cyclical.

(d) **True**   Although the severity of pain is variable, it is the cardinal symptom
of PID.

(e) **False**   Both organic and psychogenic causes of pelvic pain are unusual
after the menopause.

G 9

66 (a) **False**   Uncomplicated retroversion, without fixation, does not cause
backache.

(b) **True**   There is often premenstrual low back pain.

(c) **False**   Backache is far more likely to be due to lumbo-sacral
injuries/abnormalities.

(d) **True**   When endometriosis involves the utero-sacral ligaments, with
fixed retroversion, there is often chronic low back pain.

(e) **True**   Pregnancy often exacerbates or unmasks a lumbo-sacral cause
of back pain.

G 9

67 (a) **True**   The diagnosis is only made after biopsy, which will establish
the degree of cellular atypia, and hence the risk of malignancy
developing.

(b) **False**   The ulcers are characteristically painless.

(c) **True**   Vulval warts may be intensely itchy.

(d) **False**   Chancre is classically painless and non-irritant.

(e) **True**   In children the migration of anal threadworms may cause vulval
irritation.

G 5

68 (a) **False**   It is a *vaginal* infection.

(b) **True**   It most commonly occurs in the elderly.

(c) **True**   The degree to which atrophy occurs is very variable, and HRT
prevents this.

(d) **True**   Hyperkeratosis is the feature distinguishing it from primary
atrophy, and pruritis is often intense.

(e) **True**   Gumma formation may occur in tertiary syphilis, condylomata
lata in secondary disease and chancre in primary syphilis.

G 5

69 Bartholin's cysts:
   (a)  Should always be excised to prevent recurrence.
   (b)  Are situated on the inner side of the posterior end of the labium majus
   (c)  May become infected by gonorrhoea
   (d)  Are usually bilateral
   (e)  May be easily confused with hidradenoma

70 Carcinoma of the vulva:
   (a)  Does not ulcerate until it is advanced
   (b)  Is usually histologically anaplastic
   (c)  Spreads initially to iliac nodes via vaginal lymphatics
   (d)  Seldom involves lymph nodes at the time of presentation
   (e)  Is equally amenable to treatment by surgery and radiotherapy

71 Cervical smears:
   (a)  Are taken with a throat swab
   (b)  Should be placed in fixative immediately
   (c)  Should be taken every 10 years
   (d)  Should be followed by colposcopy if any abnormality is reported
   (e)  Should not be done in women under 21 years

72 Carcinoma *in situ* of the cervix:
   (a)  Arises from the squamo-columnar junction
   (b)  Usually becomes invasive within 3–4 years
   (c)  Causes a 'mosaic' appearance on colposcopy
   (d)  May regress spontaneously
   (e)  Merges gradually with healthy epithelium

73 Cone biopsy of the cervix:
   (a)  Should be carried out on all patients with carcinoma *in situ* unless
        hysterectomy is required for some other reason
   (b)  May cause secondary haemorrhage, with a peak incidence 14–21 days
        after the operation
   (c)  Has been carried out more frequently since the discovery of colposcopy
   (d)  Is required for symptomatic cervical erosions
   (e)  Increases the chances of caesarean section in a subsequent pregnancy

69 (a) **False** Marsupialization is the primary treatment of choice as it is a smaller operation and preserves the function of the gland.

(b) **True** A cyst in the anterior part of the labium majus may be a cyst of the canal of Nuck.

(c) **True** The vulval and vaginal skin are resistant to gonococcal infection, but Bartholin's glands, Skene's glands and the cervix may be infected.

(d) **False** It is unusual to see simultaneous bilateral cysts, but sometimes a contralateral cyst develops at a later date.

(e) **False** Hidradenoma is a small (<2 cm), solid benign tumour of sweat glands.

G 6

70 (a) **False** Ulceration is usually an early sign.

(b) **False** It is usually well differentiated.

(c) **False** Spread is to the inguinal nodes.

(d) **False** These lymph nodes are involved in 50% of cases at presentation.

(e) **False** Surrounding tissues will not tolerate effective doses of radiotherapy.

G 7

71 (a) **False** An Ayre's spatula (or variant), or cervical brush is used.

(b) **True** Air drying spoils the preparation.

(c) **False** A smear should be repeated every 3 years ideally.

(d) **False** All cases of CIN should be referred for colposcopy, but if the smear only reports 'inflammatory change', it should be repeated after treatment for any obvious inflammatory condition.

(e) **False** All sexually active women should have smears done regularly.

G 6

72 (a) **True**

(b) **False** Ten years is the mean time for invasive change.

(c) **True** This is an appearance caused by abnormal capillary patterns.

(d) **True** The exact proportion of CIN cases which will spontaneously regress is not known, but it is certainly considerable.

(e) **False** The junction between healthy and abnormal epithelium is abrupt.

G 6

73 (a) **False** Laser treatment, coagulation or some other form of 'ablation' may be employed, provided the whole ectocervix can be inspected through the colposcope.

(b) **False** The peak incidence for secondary haemorrhage is 7–10 days postoperatively.

(c) **False** Colposcopy allows selective biopsy of the affected areas to be carried out and ablation if no invasion is detected. Cone biopsy can therefore be reserved for those cases where the squamo-columnar junction is high in the endocervical canal and cannot be visualized through the colposcope.

(d) **False** These are treated by cryosurgery or coagulation.

(e) **True** Cervical stenosis (fibrosis) may prevent dilatation, although no difficulty is experienced in the majority of cases.

74 Endocervical carcinoma:
  (a)  Is usually an adenocarcinoma
  (b)  May spread directly to para-aortic nodes
  (c)  Usually causes death from local invasion before metastases become manifest
  (d)  Causes a barrel-shaped cervix
  (e)  Is usually diagnosed by means of a cone biopsy


75 Stage I cancer of the cervix:
  (a)  Is confined to the uterus
  (b)  May not be visible on clinical examination
  (c)  Has a better prognosis than stage I cancer of the endometrium
  (d)  May be associated with hydro-ureter on intravenous pyelogram
  (e)  May be treated with intracavity radiation (to provide 7000 rads at point A) and external radiotherapy


76 Radiotherapy for carcinoma of the cervix may cause:
  (a)  Vesico-vaginal fistula
  (b)  Pyometra
  (c)  Proctitis
  (d)  Acute salpingitis
  (e)  Ovarian failure


77 Carcinoma of the endometrium:
  (a)  Is very rare (less than 5%) before the menopause
  (b)  Is more common in postmenopausal women on combined oestrogen, progesterone preparations
  (c)  Is usually (over 50%) a squamous carcinoma
  (d)  Is best treated by simple hysterectomy with conservation of the ovaries in early cases
  (e)  May be diagnosed by cervical cytology in 25–30% of cases

74 (a) **False** Squamous metaplasia usually precedes malignancy.
   (b) **True** In this case, spread occurs along the ovarian lymphatics.
   (c) **True** As with ectocervical cancer, renal failure (due to ureteric obstruction) is the commonest cause of death.
   (d) **True**
   (e) **False** This is used for carcinoma *in situ* and dysplasia when an adequate colposcopically-directed biopsy is impossible, most often because the squamo-columnar junction cannot be seen.

   **G6**

75 (a) **True** Stage I may be further divided into IA and IB, but these are both confined to the cervix of the uterus.
   (b) **True** This is stage Ia.
   (c) **False** Spread to lymph nodes is more common. The 5-year corrected survival rates are 75% for stage I cancer of the cervix, and 90% for endometrial cancer.
   (d) **False** This would be classified as stage III, as staging takes into account normal pre-operative investigations.
   (e) **True** Radiation dose diminishes by the inverse square law and therefore separate internal and external doses are required to cover local lesion and pelvic nodes.

   **G 6**

76 (a) **True** But this is very rare with modern treatment in the absence of a recurrence. However, if tumour has eroded the bladder prior to treatment, this is more likely.
   (b) **True** Secretions may accumulate behind a fibrotic and stenosed cervix.
   (c) **True** This is the most common side-effect. It is treated with steroid suppositories.
   (d) **False**
   (e) **True** This is inevitable.

   **G 6**

77 (a) **False** Although the peak incidence is between the ages of 50 and 65 years, 20–25% of cases occur premenopausally.
   (b) **False** Unopposed natural (from granulosa cell tumours, polycystic ovary syndrome) or exogenous oestrogen predisposes to cancer of the endometrium; combined therapy does not. Indeed, there is now evidence that it is protective against this disease.
   (c) **False** It is usually adenocarcinoma, or occasionally, a mixture of adeno and squamous.
   (d) **False** The ovaries are a common site for metastases and oestrogen secretion activates any residual cancer cells.
   (e) **True** Although it may be picked up on cervical cytology, a negative smear does not preclude the diagnosis of endometrial carcinoma.

   **G 6**

78 Stage I carcinoma of the endometrium:
- (a) Is best managed by vaginal hysterectomy
- (b) Is confined to the uterus
- (c) Will have spread to lymph nodes in approximately 10% of patients
- (d) Is the commonest stage at the time of diagnosis
- (e) Should be treated with postoperative radiotherapy

79 Radiotherapy for cancer of the cervix:
- (a) May be curative
- (b) Has approximately the same success rate as Wertheim's hysterectomy for stage I lesions of the ectocervix
- (c) Should not be used after a Wertheim's hysterectomy
- (d) May consist of two intracavity caesium applications followed by external irradiation to the pelvic side walls
- (e) Can be repeated if the tumour recurs after the initial standard dose (5000–8000 cGy)

80 Curative radiotherapy for gynaecological malignancy:
- (a) Is dependent mainly on beta rays
- (b) May consist of intracavity radium or caesium and external radiation from supervoltage X-ray machines or cobalt
- (c) May involve intracavity cobalt
- (d) May be repeated after 2 years for a local recurrence
- (e) Is potentiated by hypoxia

81 Incontinence of urine:
- (a) Is commonly caused by prolapse
- (b) May be caused by diabetes mellitus
- (c) May be due to overflow incontinence in multiple sclerosis
- (d) May be congenital
- (e) Is best treated surgically if detrusor instability is the cause

82 Stress incontinence of urine:
- (a) Is more common in multiparous patients
- (b) Can be controlled by para-urethral pressure during vaginal examination
- (c) Can be differentiated from urge incontinence by means of a cystometrogram
- (d) Should be investigated by cystoscopy prior to surgery
- (e) May be a transient problem after delivery

78 (a) **False** This procedure should only be used if the patient is a very poor operative risk and it is usually followed by radiotherapy.

(b) **False** It is confined to the *body* of the uterus. If the cervix is involved, it is classed as stage II. This is in contrast to cancer of the cervix which is stage I provided it is confined to the uterus as a whole.

(c) **True** This is why lymph node biopsy is important.

(d) **True** Eighty per cent of cases are stage I.

(e) **False** Only cases with poor prognostic features such as deep myometrial invasion or poor differentiation should be treated in this way.

**G 6**

79 (a) **True** For example, 80–90% of stage I ectocervical cancers can be cured by this treatment.

(b) **True** This has been confirmed by several large series.

(c) **False** If cancerous lymph nodes are removed, irradiation to the pelvic side-walls is often used.

(d) **True** This is the widely used Manchester technique for cancer of the cervix.

(e) **False** The maximum dose of radiation which tissues will tolerate is 8000 cGy which cannot be repeated.

**G 6**

80 (a) **False** It is dependent on gamma rays; beta rays (electrons or positrons) and alpha particles are screened out.

(b) **True** This would be the standard radiotherapy regime for carcinoma of the cervix.

(c) **True** Cobalt is usually used for external irradiation, but a machine known as the cathetron can be used to administer intracavity cobalt irradiation.

(d) **False** This has a high risk of causing extensive necrosis and fistula formation.

(e) **False** The reverse is true.

**G 6**

81 (a) **False** It is associated with, but not caused by prolapse.

(b) **True** Diabetic neuropathy may lead to *overflow* incontinence, as with other lower motor neurone lesions.

(c) **False** This causes high pressure, urge incontinence as with other upper motor neurone lesions.

(d) **True** Occasionally a ureter may drain directly into the vagina.

(e) **False** Surgery is reserved for genuine stress incontinence.

**G 12**

82 (a) **True** Childbirth is the most important aetiological factor.

(b) **True** This is called Bonney's test.

(c) **True** Surgical operation for stress incontinence should not be done unless urodynamic tests have confirmed the diagnosis.

(d) **False** Cytoscopy has little place in the evaluation of incontinence.

(e) **True** Surgery should only be considered if incontinence persists for 3 months after delivery.

**G 12**

83 Uterovaginal prolapse:
   (a)  Is a very painful condition
   (b)  The condition is worse in the erect position
   (c)  The cervix is often elongated
   (d)  Is common in Negroes
   (e)  May cause intestinal obstruction if there is a large rectocele


84 An enterocele:
   (a)  Is a prolapse of the rectum
   (b)  May occur following a colposuspension
   (c)  Should initially be treated with a shelf pessary
   (d)  May resolve spontaneously
   (e)  Is a common cause of stress incontinence


85 Retroversion of the uterus:
   (a)  Occurs in 15% of normal women
   (b)  Is a common cause of infertility
   (c)  May be corrected by a Fothergill operation
   (d)  Is caused by heavy lifting
   (e)  Should always be corrected with a Hodge pessary in early pregnancy


86 Cystocele:
   (a)  Is a prolapse of the bladder and anterior vaginal wall
   (b)  Is common after the menopause
   (c)  Is the cause of stress incontinence of urine
   (d)  May lead to urinary infection
   (e)  Is very uncommon in nulliparous women


87 The following substances may be secreted by ovarian tumours:
   (a)  TSH
   (b)  Serotonin
   (c)  Calmodulin
   (d)  Chorionic gonadotrophin
   (e)  Vasco-active intestinal peptide

**83 (a) False** There is rarely pain, even with gross degrees of prolapse.
   **(b) True** Lying down almost always relieves prolapse.
   **(c) True** Elongation of the supravaginal cervix occurs with major degrees of uterine prolapse.
   **(d) False** It is strikingly uncommon in Negroes, despite high parity.
   **(e) False** Difficulty in defaecation may occur, but not obstruction.

**G 4**

**84 (a) False** It is a hernia of the pouch of Douglas, and therefore at a higher level than the rectum.
   **(b) True** Colposuspension alters the vaginal angle, potentially leading to hernia of the pouch of Douglas.
   **(c) False** This is only a treatment to be used in the frail and elderly, or recurrent cases.
   **(d) False** No conservative measures improve enterocele.
   **(e) False** Unless there is associated anterior vaginal prolapse, stress incontinence will not occur.

**G 4**

**85 (a) True** Provided the retroversion is mobile, it is of little clinical significance.
   **(b) False** It is only associated with infertility if there is an underlying cause such as endometriosis or chronic pelvic infection.
   **(c) False** The operation to correct retroversion is a ventrosuspension.
   **(d) False** It is either congenital, acquired following childbirth, or secondary to pelvic adhesions.
   **(e) False** A retroverted uterus only rarely becomes incarcerated in pregnancy and correction with a Hodge pessary is hardly ever indicated.

**G 4**

**86 (a) True** It may or may not be accompanied by uterine or other vaginal prolapse.
   **(b) True** Oestrogen deficiency results in atrophy of the supporting fascia.
   **(c) False** Although stress incontinence is often associated with cystocele, it is not caused by it.
   **(d) True** Stasis of urine from any cause may lead to infection.
   **(e) True** It is almost always a consequence of childbirth.

**G 4**

**87 (a) False** Thyroxine is secreted by the *Struma ovarii* of a dermoid cyst.
   **(b) True** Carcinoid syndrome may result.
   **(c) False** This is an intracellular substance. Hypercalcaemia may, however, occur due to parathormone or prostaglandin secretion.
   **(d) True** This is an important 'tumour marker' in choriocarcinoma and endodermal sinus tumour.
   **(e) False** Although these peptides may affect production of various ovarian steroids *in vivo*, they have not been shown to be produced by tumours.

**G 6**

88 The following ovarian tumours are always malignant:
   (a) Myxoma peritonei
   (b) Endodermal sinus tumour
   (c) Solid teratoma
   (d) Granulosa cell tumours
   (e) Brenner tumours

89 Mucin secreting neoplasms of the ovary:
   (a) Are usually malignant
   (b) Are usually unilocular
   (c) Can usually be differentiated from single follicular cysts by ultrasound
   (d) Are more often bilateral than other ovarian tumours
   (e) Should always be removed

90 Carcinoma of the ovary:
   (a) Has a good prognosis if the capsule of the ovary has not been penetrated
   (b) Is aggravated by oestrogens
   (c) Is classified as stage II if it has spread to the pelvic peritoneum
   (d) Typically spreads across the peritoneal cavity
   (e) Frequently causes intestinal obstruction

91 Malignant ovarian disease:
   (a) Is the commonest cause of death from cancer of the reproductive tract in Britain
   (b) Is usually (FIGO) stage IV when it is discovered
   (c) Is staged at operation, unlike cancer of the cervix, which is staged pre-operatively
   (d) Often presents with amenorrhoea in premenopausal patients
   (e) Is more common in women who have never been pregnant

92 In the management of cancer of the ovary:
   (a) Chemotherapy is more effective than with other epithelial tumours
   (b) Progesterone administration may cause a temporary remission
   (c) Extensive surgery has no place in (FIGO) stage III carcinoma
   (d) Dysgerminomas are effectively treated by radiotherapy
   (e) Radiotherapy has a very limited place

88 **(a) False** Although spread of benign mucinous cells through the peritoneal cavity is a very serious disorder leading to cachexia, it cannot be regarded as a malignant tumour.
   **(b) True** Potentially this is the most malignant tumour in the human body, but the prognosis has been transformed by chemotherapy.
   **(c) False** If mature tissues predominate, it is benign.
   **(d) False** Only about 30% are malignant. Malignant potential cannot however be reliably predicted from histological appearance.
   **(e) False** These are nearly always benign.

G 6

89 **(a) False** Only 5–10% are malignant.
   **(b) False**
   **(c) True** The loculi show up on ultrasound.
   **(d) False** Only 5% are bilateral, whilst 50% of serous cystadenocarcinomas are bilateral.
   **(e) True** Unlike simple functional cysts, all neoplasms of the ovary should be removed to exclude malignancy and prevent complications such as torsion or rupture.

G 6

90 **(a) True** Unfortunately ovarian cancer is seldom detected at this early stage. Occasionally, however, such stage Ia tumours are discovered by chance at laparotomy for other reasons.
   **(b) False** It is seldom, if ever, hormone responsive.
   **(c) True** Stage II implies spread within the pelvis.
   **(d) True** This is the most common mode of spread.
   **(e) True** This is a frequent terminal complication.

G 6

91 **(a) True** It is not, however, the commonest malignancy of the reproductive organs.
   **(b) False** It is usually stage III. However, this denotes abdominal spread beyond the pelvic capacity and the prognosis is usually poor.
   **(c) True** Laparotomy is the only method of absolutely determining the extent of spread.
   **(d) False** Only the rare androgen secreting tumours cause amenorrhoea at an early stage.
   **(e) True** There is an association with low or nil parity.

G 6

92 **(a) True**
   **(b) False** Endometrial carcinoma may have hormone receptors and respond temporarily to progesterone treatment.
   **(c) False** Removal of the bulk of the tumour mass increases the response rate of chemotherapy.
   **(d) True** They are sensitive to radiotherapy in the same way as seminomas, which they resemble histologically.
   **(e) True** It is useful for the rare dysgerminoma, and rarely for stage II disease.

G 6

93 Midline incisions are inferior to lower transverse incisions for gynaecological operations in the following respects:
  (a) Exposure is less adequate
  (b) Incisional hernia is more common
  (c) Dehiscence of the scar is more likely
  (d) Wound haematoma is more common
  (e) The cosmetic result is worse

94 The abdominal approach for hysterectomy has the following advantages over vaginal hysterectomy:
  (a) It causes less postoperative pain
  (b) The ovaries may be removed more easily if an unexpected endometrial cancer is discovered
  (c) A large uterus is easily removed
  (d) Prolapse can be repaired more adequately by plicating the uterosacral ligaments
  (e) Postoperative recovery is more rapid

95 Anterior colporrhaphy:
  (a) May cause temporary retention of urine
  (b) Is used in the treatment of stress incontinence
  (c) Is frequently combined with vaginal hysterectomy
  (d) Should be avoided in patients with urge incontinence
  (e) Should not be carried out until childbearing is complete

96 Dilatation and curettage (D & C):
  (a) Should be carried out in all patients with menorrhagia
  (b) Should be carried out for all patients with postmenopausal bleeding
  (c) Should be recommended for all patients with breakthrough bleeding on oral contraception.
  (d) May be helpful in the diagnosis of ectopic pregnancy
  (e) Is an essential investigation for subfertility

**93 (a) False** It is better and the incision may easily be extended.
  **(b) True** The rectus sheath should be repaired with a non-absorbable material to lower the incidence of this complication after midline incisions.
  **(c) True** Dehiscence of low transverse incisions is almost unknown.
  **(d) False** The large exposed areas behind the rectus sheath and on the surface of the rectus abdominus muscles predispose to haematoma formation. The wound is often drained for this reason.
  **(e) True** The incision cuts across Lange's lines, and therefore leaves a wider scar.

G 13

**94 (a) False** However, if posterior repair is carried out at the time of vaginal hysterectomy, considerable pain will be experienced.
  **(b) True** Some surgeons perform a D & C to exclude frank malignancy before performing vaginal hysterectomy.
  **(c) True** Removal of a large uterus vaginally often requires morcellation of the uterus.
  **(d) False** Vaginal hysterectomy with suture of the vault to the cardinal and uterosacral ligaments together with anterior and posterior repair (if required) is the standard operation for prolapse.
  **(e) False** Many patients are ready to return home 2–3 days after vaginal hysterectomy.

G 13

**95 (a) True** Routine postoperative catheterization, preferably with a supra-pubic catheter, is often used for this purpose.
  **(b) True** However, colposuspension procedures have a higher success rate.
  **(c) True**
  **(d) True** It may make matters worse.
  **(e) False** Most surgeons would however recommend delivery by caesarean section after successful anterior colporrhapy.

G 13

**96 (a) False** If periods are heavy but still regular and the patient is less than, say, 35 years of age, an endometrial cancer is so unlikely that D & C is not mandatory.
  **(b) True** Even if another cause, such as atrophic vaginitis, is discovered.
  **(c) False** It should, however, be carried out if this persists after changing oral contraceptive.
  **(d) True** Discovery of products of conception almost eliminates an ectopic pregnancy, while the presence of decidua with no trophoblast makes the diagnosis more likely.
  **(e) False** Ovulation can now be diagnosed biochemically and a routine endometrial culture for tuberculosis is not essential in Britain.

G 13

# PART II

# OBSTETRICS

97 For a woman's menstrual dates to be reliable in predicting gestational age:
   (a) The cycle must be 28 days long
   (b) She must have discontinued the oral contraceptive pill at least 1 month before the last menstrual period
   (c) She must have had an ultrasound examination in early pregnancy that confirms the dates
   (d) There should have been no bleeding in early pregnancy
   (e) She must not be carrying twins

98 The following statements are true of tests used in prenatal diagnosis:
   (a) Biochemical tests on maternal blood are superior to maternal age alone as a screening test for Down's syndrome
   (b) Maternal serum alphafetoprotein is a diagnostic test for neural tube defects
   (c) Chorionic villus sampling has a lower pregnancy loss rate than amniocentesis
   (d) Tests using DNA technology can be performed on amniocentesis specimens
   (e) Chorionic villus sampling can only be performed before 12 weeks' gestation

99 By the time a fetus is mature it is usual for:
   (a) Meconium to have been passed
   (b) Pulmonary surfactant to have been produced
   (c) The ductus arteriosus to have closed
   (d) Hepatic glucuronyl transferase system to be adequate
   (e) Fetal haemoglobin to be 16–20 g/100 ml

100 The denominator (indicator):
   (a) Is the occiput in a flexed cephalic presentation
   (b) Is the fetal part most closely related to the symphysis pubis
   (c) Of a face presentation is the submento-bregmatic diameter
   (d) Of a breech presentation is the sacrum
   (e) Is used to determine the position

101 The fetal head:
   (a) Engages by the mento-vertical diameter in face presentations
   (b) Has a suboccipito-bregmatic diameter of 10.5 cm
   (c) Contains an anterior fontanelle immediately behind the bregma
   (d) Has one occipital and two frontal bones
   (e) May be felt abdominally after engagement has taken place

**97 (a) False**   If a woman's cycle length is consistently longer or shorter, allowance can be made in the calculation.

**(b) True**   Ovulation is often delayed in the first few menstrual cycles.

**(c) False**   An early scan may confirm or refute menstrual dates.

**(d) True**   Bleeding from a threatened abortion may be confused with a menstrual period.

**(e) False**   Although the uterine size will be greater, and labour is likely to be pre-term, this does not affect the gestational age.

OB 2

**98 (a) True**   Sixty to 70% of Down's fetuses will be picked up by biochemical screening, compared with 30–40% by age alone.

**(b) False**   It is a *screening* test, requiring confirmation by ultrasound (or amniotic fluid AFP estimation).

**(c) False**   Amniocentesis prior to 13 weeks carries a higher pregnancy loss rate than CVS, but 'standard' 16-week amniocentesis is safer.

**(d) True**   Amplification of DNA can be used, but the larger amounts of DNA in chorion villus samples makes this the chosen method of sampling for such techniques.

**(e) False**   It can be carried out between 8 and 14 weeks, but there is a risk of fetal damage if performed earlier than 10 weeks.

OB 2

**99 (a) False**   If meconium is passed before birth, it is usually a sign of fetal distress.

**(b) True**   This is normally present from the 32nd to the 34th week of gestation.

**(c) False**   It usually closes some time after birth.

**(d) False**   The inadequacy of this enzyme system is the cause of physiological jaundice.

**(e) True**

**100 (a) True**

**(b) False**   It would be in a direct occipito-anterior position but is not necessarily so. For example, it is the part most closely related to the sacro-iliac joint in an occipito-posterior position.

**(c) False**   The chin is the denominator.

**(d) True**

**(e) True**   The position describes the relationship of the denominator to the maternal pelvis.

OB 4 & 5

**101 (a) False**   The mento-vertical diameter is associated with brow presentations and, as it measures 13 cm, engagement cannot take place in the term fetus.

**(b) False**   This is the diameter which engages when the head is well flexed and measures 9.5 cm.

**(c) False**   The bregma is the point in the middle of the anterior fontanelle.

**(d) True**

**(e) True**   After engagement, two-fifths, one-fifth or none of the head may be felt abdominally.

OB 4 & 5

102 The following terms are appropriate:
  (a) Lie: cephalic
  (b) Position: flexed
  (c) Station: at the level of the spines
  (d) Engagement: two-fifths palpable
  (e) Presenting part: shoulder

103 In the fetal circulation:
  (a) Oxygenated blood travels along the umbilical arteries
  (b) The fetal lungs are by-passed by means of the ductus venosus
  (c) The foramen ovale connects the two atria
  (d) Most of the blood entering the right atrium flows into the left atrium
  (e) The blood in the descending aorta is more desaturated than that in the ascending aorta

104 Compared with maternal venous blood, blood in the umbilical vein has:
  (a) Smaller red blood cells
  (b) A higher haemoglobin concentration
  (c) A higher oxygen saturation
  (d) A higher oxygen content
  (e) A higher oxygen partial pressure

105 Maternal blood flow to the placenta:
  (a) Reaches about 1000 ml per min by the end of pregnancy
  (b) Is affected by posture
  (c) Is completely obstructed during the peak of strong contractions
  (d) Is reduced in pre-eclampsia
  (e) Is increased by inspiration of 100% oxygen

106 By means of real-time ultrasound examination:
  (a) Pregnancy can usually be detected 5 weeks after the last menstrual period
  (b) The fetal heart cannot be seen until 10 weeks after the last period
  (c) Placenta praevia can be reliably demonstrated at the 16th week of pregnancy
  (d) The biparietal diameter can be measured reliably after the 12th week of pregnancy
  (e) A reliable estimate of gestational age can be made in the third trimester

102 (a) **False** Cephalic describes presentation.
   (b) **False** Flexion describes the attitude.
   (c) **True** Indicates that the presenting part has reached the ischial spines.
   (d) **True** For descriptive purposes the fetal head is divided into fifths.
   (e) **True** The shoulder presents with a transverse lie.

OB 2

103 (a) **False** Deoxygenated blood is returned to the placenta via the umbilical arteries.
   (b) **False** It is the ductus arteriosus.
   (c) **True** Blood passes from the right to the left atrium.
   (d) **True** Blood from the IVC passes through the foramen ovale.
   (e) **True** Admixture of blood from the ductus arteriosus causes the lower oxygen saturation.

OB 1

104 (a) **False** Fetal red cells are larger than those of the adult.
   (b) **True** Eighteen compared with 12 g/100 ml.
   (c) **True** Eighty compared with 40%.
   (d) **True** Twenty-one compared with 10 ml $O_2$ per 100 ml blood.
   (e) **False** The higher haemoglobin concentration and greater oxygen affinity of fetal haemoglobin result in a higher oxygen content despite lower partial pressure.

OB 1

105 (a) **True**
   (b) **True** Pressure of the uterus on the interior vena cava in the supine position obstructs venous return from the uterus.
   (c) **True** Venules in the myometrium are completely occluded by surrounding muscle fibres.
   (d) **True** This is an important ccomponent of the pathophysiology of pre-eclampsia and may even be the primary event.
   (e) **False** There is some evidence that it may be decreased, but none that it is increased. Oxygen administration nevertheless is a beneficial temporary measure in fetal distress.

OB 1

106 (a) **True** Transvaginal ultrasound detects the gestation sac by 5 weeks, i.e. 1 week earlier than abdominal ultrasound.
   (b) **False** It can normally be demonstrated at 6–7 weeks by vaginal ultrasound, although 10–12 weeks are necessary for detection by Doppler.
   (c) **False** Five to 15% of all pregnancies will have an apparently low placenta at this gestation, as the lower segment has not yet formed to any appreciable degree.
   (d) **True** It is measurable accurately from 12 weeks' gestation – crown–rump length is most accurate between 8 and 12 weeks.
   (e) **False** This is the result of the wide range of fetal size for given gestational age at this stage of pregnancy, and the slow rate of growth compared to the inherent range of error of the technique.

OB 2

107 The following ultrasonic measurements may be used to confirm or establish gestational age:
    (a) Crown–rump length
    (b) Biparietal diameter
    (c) Nuchal pad thickness
    (d) Gestational sac volume
    (e) Yolk sac volume

108 Ultrasound:
    (a) Only applies to sound in the megahertz range
    (b) Will detect an intra-uterine pregnancy before a beta HCG test becomes positive
    (c) Measurements can be used to establish gestational age in the third trimester
    (d) Localization of the placenta at 16–20 weeks is a specific test for placenta praevia in the third trimester
    (e) Is used in antenatal cardiotocography

109 The fetus:
    (a) Is recognizably human at 12 weeks of gestation
    (b) Usually weighs over a kilogram at 28 weeks
    (c) Develops recognizable external genitalia at 14 weeks
    (d) Can survive hypoxia for longer than an adult
    (e) Will develop anaemia if the mother is iron-deficient
    (f) Is most vulnerable to teratogenic agents between 10 and 12 weeks

110 During the development of ovarian follicles:
    (a) The first polar body is extruded before ovulation
    (b) Meiosis is resumed 1 week before ovulation
    (c) The ovum is extruded at the peak of the LH surge
    (d) Progesterone secretion starts to increase before ovulation
    (e) Granulosa cells in the corpus luteum are responsible for steroidogenesis

111 Biochemical screening for chromosomal abnormalities:
    (a) Can provide risk estimates for trisomy 18
    (b) Includes HCG which has a low level in association with Down's syndrome
    (c) Is most accurate when femur length is used to assess gestational age
    (d) Can be an indicator of other poor fetal outcomes
    (e) Does not take maternal age into account

107 (a) **True**   This is most accurate between 7 and 12 weeks.

(b) **True**   This is the most appropriate measurement between 14 and 20 weeks.

(c) **False**   A thick nuchal pad is a predictor of possible Down's syndrome.

(d) **True**   This is useful in very early pregnancy.

(d) **False**   The yolk sac is too small and does not correlate well with gestational age.

OB 2

108 (a) **False**   The human ear only detects sound up to 20 kHz. Medical ultrasound uses 1–10 MHz.

(b) **False**   Even the most sophisticated ultrasound equipment will not detect the presence of a pregnancy sac until 4–5 weeks, whereas $\beta$HCG is detectable even before the missed period.

(c) **False**   The range of measurements of fetal size in the third trimester is much too wide to be useful for this purpose.

(d) **False**   An apparently low-lying placenta at 16–20 weeks will only predict placenta praevia in a very small proportion of cases.

(e) **True**   The external transducer uses ultrasound to record fetal heart rate.

OB 2

109 (a) **True**

(b) **True**   The average fetal weight at 28 weeks is 1100 g.

(c) **True**   Modern ultrasound equipment will often permit diagnosis of sex at 14 weeks.

(d) **True**

(e) **False**   Fetal serum iron concentration is higher than maternal, and will be maintained at the expense of the mother.

(f) **False**   The most critical period is in the early first trimester when most organogenesis occurs.

OB 1

110 (a) **True**   The primary oocyte divides by meiosis while still in the ovary.

(b) **False**   It is resumed 36–48 h after the peak and 36 h after the start of the LH surge.

(c) **False**   Ovulation occurs 12 h after the peak and 36 h after the start of the LH surge.

(d) **True**   It does not reach a peak level until 7 days after ovulation, but begins to rise well before

(e) **True**   They become granulosa lutein cells, and provide steriods.

OB 1

111 (a) **True**   Although the 'Triple test' is designed for screening for Down's syndrome, a low level of HCG is a marker for trisomy 18.

(b) **False**   HCG is raised in Down's syndrome.

(c) **False**   Femur length is shorter in Down's fetuses, hence reducing the sensitivity of the test.

(d) **True**   Elevated AFP levels indicate increased risk of neural tube defects and other abnormalities.

(e) **False**   Maternal age and weight are included in the risk calculation.

OB 2

112 The luteal phase of the menstrual cycle is associated with:
  (a) High progesterone levels
  (b) High LH levels
  (c) Low basal body temperature
  (d) Implantation
  (e) Rising FSH levels

113 During normal pregnancy:
  (a) Estradiol is the principal circulating oestrogen
  (b) The blood pressure falls in the second trimester
  (c) Blood flow to the liver and kidneys increases by over 25%
  (d) The pressure of the uterus on the diaphragm reduces the tidal volume and causes dyspnoea
  (e) The ureters dilate due to obstruction and increased intraluminal pressure

114 Fibroids in pregnancy:
  (a) Are a recognized cause of obstructed labour
  (b) Should be removed by myomectomy during pregnancy
  (c) Should be removed by myomectomy at caesarean section
  (d) Are likely to regress after the pregnancy
  (e) May cause acute abdominal pain

115 Retroversion of the uterus in pregnancy:
  (a) Is a common cause of recurrent abortion
  (b) Causes acute retention of urine at the 10th week
  (c) Should be corrected by the insertion of a Hodge pessary
  (d) Usually corrects itself spontaneously after the 12th week
  (e) Is often associated with stress incontinence

116 In ectopic pregnancy:
  (a) Bleeding precedes pain
  (b) Shoulder tip pain is an important symptom
  (c) The isthmus of the tube is the commonest site of implantation
  (d) The incidence is greater in women wearing intra-uterine devices
  (e) Ultrasonic scan is of no help in diagnosis

112 (a) **True** It reaches a peak at mid-luteal phase.
   (b) **False** The LH peak occurs prior to ovulation.
   (c) **False** The basal temperature rises after ovulation.
   (d) **True** The blastocyst starts to implant 7 days after ovulation.
   (e) **False** The FSH level rises in the follicular phase.

                                                       **OB 1**

113 (a) **False** Estriol is the principal oestrogen.
   (b) **True** The diastolic pressure is reduced in both the first and second trimester
   (c) **False** Blood flow to the kidneys increases by 30% but splanchnic and hepatic flow is unchanged.
   (d) **False** Tidal volume is increased due to the effect of progesterone on the respriatory centre.
   (e) **False** Intraluminal pressure is low; dilation is due to the smooth muscle relaxant effect of progesterone.

                                                        **OB 1**

114 (a) **True** Fibroids situated in the pelvis may obstruct labour, but the growing uterus usually raises them out of the pelvis.
   (b) **False** There is a high risk of abortion and haemorrhage if myomectomy is attempted in pregnancy
   (c) **False** Again, dangerous haemorrhage may occur.
   (d) **True**
   (e) **True** Degeneration of fibroids is common in pregnancy, causing severe pain.

                                                        **OB 3**

115 (a) **False** This misconception was abandoned many years ago.
   (b) **False** It causes retention between the 12th and 16th week.
   (c) **False** This is not generally necessary as the retroversion corrects itself.
   (d) **True** Only very rarely does incarceration occur.
   (e) **False** If incarceration occurs, urinary retention with overflow incontinence occurs.

                                                        **OB 3**

116 (a) **False** Pain usually precedes bleeding.
   (b) **True** Blood tracks up the paracolic gutters to the diaphragm where it causes referred pain.
   (c) **False** The ampulla is the commonest site.
   (d) **True** The copper containing devices probably interfere with tubal motility and ciliary function.
   (e) **False** Tubal pregnancy is often identified on transvaginal ultrasonic scan, and the scan is also helpful in excluding an intra-uterine pregnancy when the beta HCG is positive.

                                                        **OB 3**

117 Complications of hydatidiform mole include:
  (a) Hyperemesis gravidarum
  (b) Malignant change
  (c) Haemorrhage
  (d) Diabetes insipidus
  (e) Development of ovarian cysts

118 First trimester abortion may be due to:
  (a) Inadequate oestrogen production
  (b) Chromosome abnormality of the fetus
  (c) Incompetence of the internal cervical os
  (d) Maternal diabetes
  (e) Cytotoxic drugs

119 In eclampsia:
  (a) Large doses of intravenous sedation are given
  (b) Caesarean section must be carried out, whether the fetus is dead or alive
  (c) Hypotensive drugs should not be used
  (d) Ergometrine should be avoided in the third stage of labour
  (e) Urinary output is increased

120 In pre-eclamptic toxaemia:
  (a) There is an increase in extracellular sodium
  (b) Proteinurea is the earliest sign
  (c) Serum uric acid levels tend to decrease
  (d) The hepatic lesion shows patchy haemorrhage and necrosis
  (e) There is disturbance of the clotting mechanism

121 There is an increased risk of developing pre-eclampsia with:
  (a) Increasing maternal age
  (b) High parity
  (c) Hydatidiform mole
  (d) Maternal cardiac disease
  (e) Diabetes

117 (a) **True**   This is thought to be due to the excessive production of chorionic gondadotrophin.
(b) **True**   Two to 10% progress to choriocarcinoma, the incidence varying in different parts of the world.
(c) **True**   Expulsion of the mole or surgical evacuation may be associated with haemorrhage.
(d) **False**   There is no association with diabetes insipidus (or mellitus).
(e) **True**   Theca lutein cysts of the ovary may develop due to stimulation by chorionic gonadotrophin.

**OB 3**

118 (a) **False**   This theory has been discredited.
(b) **True**   Some 60% of abortion material has been found to be chromosomally abnormal.
(c) **False**   Cervical incompetence causes mid-trimester abortion.
(d) **True**   Poorly controlled diabetes may cause abortion.
(e) **True**   For this reason, cytotoxic drugs would not knowingly be given in pregnancy.

**OB 3**

119 (a) **True**   Magnesium sulphate infusion is increasingly accepted as the sedative of choice.
(b) **False**   If the fetus is dead or the cervix very favourable, induction of labour may be attempted.
(c) **False**   Hypotensives are used to reduce the risk of cerebral haemorrhage.
(d) **True**   The vasocostrictor effect raises the blood pressure; syntocinon is preferable.
(e) **False**   There is oliguria (which may progress to renal failure).

**OB 3**

120 (a) **True**   There is retention of both water and sodium.
(b) **False**   Weight gain, oedema and hypertension usually precede proteinurea.
(c) **False**   Levels increase as a result of an alteration in renal tubular function.
(d) **True**   Characteristic red and yellow focal areas are seen.
(e) **True**   There is a fall in platelets, and an increased level of fibrin degradation products.

**OB 3**

121 (a) **True**   It is more common in women over 35 years.
(b) **False**   It is more common in primagravidae.
(c) **True**   The hypertension is severe and it often starts as early as 16–20 weeks.
(d) **False**   There is no relation with cardiac disease.
(e) **True**   This is presumed to be due to diabetic vascular disease.

**OB 3**

122 Coagulation failure is an important complication of:
  (a) Placenta praevia
  (b) Abruptio placentae
  (c) Amniotic fluid embolus
  (d) Gram-negative septicaemia
  (e) Uterine rupture

123 The following may cause intra-uterine death of the fetus:
  (a) Diabetes mellitus
  (b) Respiratory distress syndrome (RDS)
  (c) Hydrops fetalis
  (d) A sudden emotional shock to the mother
  (e) Syphilis

124 Impaired fetal growth:
  (a) Is 'symmetrical' if the fetal head and abdomen are equally reduced in size
  (b) Has long-term effects on postnatal growth if it is 'asymmetrical' in type
  (c) Is rarely associated with hypoxia and acidosis if it is symmetrical in type
  (d) May be due to maternal heroin abuse if 'symmetrical' in type
  (e) May be assessed with a single ultrasound examination in the third trimester

125 Antenatal management of an asymmetrically small fetus should include:
  (a) Ultrasound examination to measure growth
  (b) Maternal scoring of fetal movements
  (c) Serial measurement of plasma oestradiol or human placental lactogen (HPL)
  (d) Cardiotocography
  (e) Fetal scalp sampling

126 In cases of intra-uterine death:
  (a) Induction of labour should always begin immediately
  (b) It is always best to give immediate, detailed information as to the possible cause
  (c) The baby must always be shown to the parents
  (d) It is important to discuss contraception prior to hospital discharge
  (e) Lactation is likely to occur and become distressing

**122 (a) False** There is straightforward haemorrhage in this condition.
   **(b) True** Disseminated intravascular coagulation is thought to occur possibly as a result of thromboplastin release from the placental site.
   **(c) True** There is widespread disseminated intravascular coagulation.
   **(d) True** Endotoxins stimulate the clotting mechanism along with many other systems such as complement and kinins. This is particularly likely to occur in pregnancy.
   **(e) False** Although uterine rupture may lead to shock, and collapse, DIC does not usually occur.

**OB 5**

**123 (a) True** Poorly controlled diabetes may lead to sudden fetal death.
   **(b) False** This is a cause of neonatal death.
   **(c) True** Severe haemolytic disease may lead to hydrops fetalis and fetal death.
   **(d) False** This only occurs in fiction!
   **(e) True** Untreated syphilis is one of the rare causes.

**OB 3**

**124 (a) True** All parts of fetal growth velocity are affected equally.
   **(b) False** 'Asymetrical' growth reflects an inadequate supply of nutrients (and oxygen in more severe cases) to the fetus. Catch-up growth will therefore occur postnatally.
   **(c) True** It is more likely to be constitutional or associated with a specific fetal problem (e.g. chromosomal abnormality).
   **(d) True** Heroin abuse, alcohol and smoking all cause symmetrical growth impairment.
   **(e) False** Serial ultrasound measurement are necessary to confirm impaired fetal growth.

**OB 2**

**125 (a) True** A fall-off in growth rate may prompt delivery.
   **(b) True** Reduction in fetal movement may indicate fetal hypoxia.
   **(c) False** Measurement of placental hormones is now known to be an insensitive and misleading test of fetal wellbeing.
   **(d) True** This is the most informative of the biophysical tests of fetal wellbeing.
   **(e) False** This can only be done in labour, but in some circumstances cordocentesis may be appropriate.

**OB 2**

**126 (a) False** Unless there are good medical reasons to induce labour, parents can be given time to take in the news.
   **(b) False** Parents are shocked and unable to receive detailed information.
   **(c) False** This should be offered, but some parents will not want to see the baby for personal or religious/cultural reasons.
   **(d) True** This is difficult and often forgotten, but should be discussed, as it is usually wise to have an interval prior to the next pregnancy.
   **(e) True** The milk often 'comes in' after the mother has left hospital, and she needs to be warned of this and offered suppression of lactation.

**OB 3**

uterine death of the fetus occurs in the third trimester:
arean section should be carried out to deliver the fetus
e is a tendency to thrombo-embolism
re is a danger of anaerobic infection
ctation will not occur after delivery
(b, ne birth of the baby must be registered

128 Polyhydramnios is associated with the following:
(a) Chorio-angioma of the placenta
(b) Maternal diabetes
(c) Hydatidiform mole
(d) Hydrops fetalis
(e) Intra-uterine growth retardation of the fetus

129 Oligohydramnios is associated with the following fetal conditions:
(a) Tracheo-oesophageal fistula
(b) Talipes
(c) Potter's syndrome
(d) Intra-uterine growth retardation
(e) Anencephaly

130 The incidence of multiple pregnancy is increased:
(a) In people of Negro race
(b) In women treated with bromocriptine for infertility
(c) In women treated by *in vitro* fertilization
(d) With advancing maternal age
(e) First pregnancies

131 In twin delivery:
(a) The first twin is at greater risk than the second
(b) Labour usually occurs before term
(c) Epidural analgesia is best avoided
(d) There is an increased risk of post-partum haemorrhage
(e) The commonest presentation is one cephalic, one breech

132 Ante-partum haemorrhage:
(a) Is defined as 'bleeding from the genital tract in pregnancy'.
(b) May be complicated by hypofibrinogenaemia
(c) Requires assessment by vaginal examination
(d) May be caused by cervical carcinoma
(e) Is always painless

# OBSTETRICS – *Answers*

127 **(a) False** Vaginal delivery is much to be preferred.
    **(b) False** Hypofibrinogenaemia may occur resulting in failure of blood coagulation.
    **(c) True** Once the membranes have ruptured there is an ideal culture medium for anaerobic organisms.
    **(d) False** Suppression of lactation should be considered.
    **(e) True** It must be registered as a stillbirth.

OB 3

128 **(a) True** This is a rare 'fetal' cause.
    **(b) True** This is likely if the diabetes is poorly controlled, and it is probably due to fetal polyuria.
    **(c) False** The uterus is filled with molar tissue.
    **(d) True** This is often the case in severe rhesus iso-immunization.
    **(e) False** It is often associated with oligohydramnios.

OB 3

129 **(a) False** This causes hydramnios due to failure of swallowing.
    **(b) True** Limb deformations occur because of local pressure.
    **(c) True** Renal agenesis results in lack of liquor.
    **(d) True** Poor placental function is associated with oligohydramnios.
    **(e) False** Often associated with hydramnios due to inability of fetus to swallow.

OB 3

130 **(a) True** In some West African tribes, the incidence is 1:30 (cf. 1:90 in Caucasians).
    **(b) False** Bromocriptine does not induce multiple ovulation.
    **(c) True** The replacement of several embryos leads to a greater risk of multiple pregnancy.
    **(d) True** Binovular twinning increases with age up to about 40 years.
    **(e) False** It is commonest in multigravid women.

OB 3

131 **(a) False** Fetal mortality and morbidity is greater in the second twin.
    **(b) True** Over-distension of the uterus leads to pre-term labour.
    **(c) False** Epidural analgesia is ideal, in preparation for any second-stage difficulties.
    **(d) True** The larger placental site is probably the aetiological factor.
    **(e) False** The commonest presentation is cephalic–cephalic (45%).

OB 3

132 **(a) False** It is bleeding from the genital tract after fetal viability (*ca.* 24 weeks).
    **(a) True** This occurs in placental abruption, due to release of thromboplastins from the placenta.
    **(c) False** Vaginal examination is dangerous until placenta praevia has been ruled out.
    **(d) True** This is an 'incidental' cause of APH.
    **(e) False** Placental abruption is usually painful, whilst bleeding from placenta praevia is painless.

OB 3

ıesus disease iso-immunization anti-D should be given to rhesus
,men:

, 72 h of.delivery of a rhesus positive child
are known to have rhesus antibodies, within 72 h of delivery
ɔwing a termination of pregnancy, even when the father is known to be
.erozygous
- (d) When an external cephalic version has been performed
- (e) When an ultrasonic scan has been performed

134 In rhesus iso-immunization the following tests may be helpful:
- (a) Rhesus antibody titre in liquor
- (b) Liquor bilirubin level
- (c) Maternal serum bilirubin
- (d) Direct Coombs' test on cord blood
- (e) Rhesus genotype of father

135 Maternal mortality:
- (a) Now stands at a rate of less than 0.1 per thousand total births
- (b) Does not include deaths from therapeutic abortion
- (c) Must be reported to the Coroner
- (d) Is subjected to a Confidential Enquiry
- (e) Is most often caused by sepsis

136 Post-partum haemorrhage:
- (a) Is defined as a blood loss of 1 litre
- (b) Is less likely if oxytocics are administered routinely in the third stage of labour
- (c) Is 'primary' if it occurs within the first 12 h
- (d) Is common after both placenta praevia and abruptio placentae
- (e) May require manual removal of the placenta

137 The following are always indications for caesarean section:
- (a) Hydrocephalus
- (b) Grade 4 placenta praevia
- (c) Abruptio placentae
- (d) Untreated stage Ib cancer of the cervix
- (e) Active primary genital herpes

133 **(a) True** If there has been feto-maternal haemorrhage at delivery this will prevent iso-immunization.

**(b) False** Giving anti-D once there are rhesus antibodies is a useless exercise.

**(c) True** A heterozygous father has a 50% chance of producing a rhesus positive offspring.

**(d) True** The trauma of version may produce feto-maternal haemorrhage.

**(e) False** There is insufficient trauma to cause feto-maternal haemorrhage.

**OB 3**

134 **(a) False** Rhesus antibody titre in *maternal blood* is done periodically to assess the likelihood of the fetus being affected.

**(b) True** This is usually done spectrophotometrically on liquor obtained at an amniocentesis.

**(c) False** The maternal bilirubin is not altered.

**(d) True** This test confirms whether the baby is affected.

**(e) True** If the partner is heterozygous, there is a 50% chance that the offspring will not be affected.

**OB 9**

135 **(a) True** The rate has fallen to this level from 4 per 1000 in 1928.

**(b) False** Deaths from abortion, both spontaneous and therapeutic are included.

**(c) False** The same regulations relate to reporting to the coroner as with any kind of death.

**(d) True** This is a national audit which has done much to focus attention on areas where standards of care can be improved.

**(e) False** Hypertension and pulmonary embolus are the biggest causes of death.

**OB 11**

136 **(a) False** Five hundred to 600 ml is a more usual figure.

**(b) True** This has been confirmed by several randomized trials.

**(c) False** Secondary post-partum haemorrhage occurs after 24 h.

**(d) True** In placenta praevia, large placental vessels are surrounded by relatively thin and poorly contractile lower uterine segment which is unable to provide effective occlusive power. In abruptio placenta, **(i)** the bruised 'couvelaire' uterus tends to remain hypotonic, and **(ii)** consumptive coagulopathy is often present.

**(e) True** If bleeding continues and the placenta remains undelivered, manual removal should be performed under general or epidural anaesthesia.

**OB 2**

137 **(a) False** The hydrocephalus can usually be decompressed transcervically or by ultrasound directed transcutaneous methods.

**(b) True** This is the safest method of delivery, even if the fetus is dead.

**(c) False** The baby is often dead in these cases and vaginal delivery is preferable if labour progresses rapidly.

**(d) True** Cervical dilatation (and vaginal delivery) disseminates cancer cells.

**(e) True** Primary genital herpes may infect the infant during birth. This causes encephalitis and has a high mortality.

**OB 8**

138 During vaginal breech delivery:
  (a) Episiotomy should be carried out immediately before delivery of the head
  (b) There is a risk that the 'after coming' head may be retained by a rim of cervix
  (c) Traction on the anterior groin should be used if the breech does not enter the pelvis in the second stage
  (d) Løvset's manoeuvre should always be carried out
  (e) Pre-existing hypoxia is no more dangerous than it would be with vertex delivery

139 Obstructed labour:
  (a) Always develops before full dilatation of the cervix
  (b) Can usually be predicted before the onset of labour
  (c) Is more common in developed countries
  (d) Is inevitable in a term fetus with persistent mento-posterior position
  (e) Can often be overcome by means of craniotomy if the fetus is dead

140 The following are correct associations:
  (a) Anencephaly – face presentation
  (b) Advancing maternal age – Turner's syndrome
  (c) Hydatidiform mole – pre-eclampsia
  (d) Diabetes mellitus – neonatal hyperglycaemia
  (e) Precipitate labour – post-partum haemorrhage

141 Fetal tachycardia:
  (a) May be the result of previous maternal thyrotoxicosis
  (b) Usually has a good prognosis if baseline variability is retained
  (c) Is more common after prolonged rupture of the membranes
  (d) Seldom exceeds 200 beats per min
  (e) May occur in severe rhesus disease

138 (a) **False** It should be carried out when the buttock distends the perineum.
    (b) **True** This is particularly likely with a premature or footling breech.
    (c) **False** If the breech remains high, caesarean section is indicated. This suggests pelvic disproportion and the head is likely to be obstructed or damaged if the breech is delivered vaginally.
    (d) **False** This is carried out for nuchal displacement of the arms.
    (e) **False** A degree of asphyxia is inevitable in vaginal breech delivery because the cord is obstructed once the chest enters the pelvis. This can only be tolerated if the fetus is well oxygenated prior to delivery.

        **OB 5**

139 (a) **False** In most cases of obstructed labour, cervical dilatation is slow and full dilation may never occur. In others, the patient proceeds to full dilation without delay, and is then unable to deliver the fetus.
    (b) **False** In some cases, for example those with a bony deformity of the pelvis, this can be predicted. In most cases, however, it is impossible to predict the outcome of labour with any accuracy.
    (c) **False** The mean pelvic size is smaller in non-developed countries.
    (d) **True** The mento-posterior position usually results in a rotation through three-eighths of a circle which permits delivery in the mento-anterior position. If this fails to occur, there is no mechanism for delivery and manual rotation, Kielland's forceps or caesarean section is required.
    (e) **True** Craniotomy will be effective if the fetus is presenting by the vertex; more complex destructive operations or caesarean section are required for an impacted, dead transverse lie.

        **OB 5**

140 (a) **True** The abnormal head faces downwards, making face presentation likely.
    (b) **False** Unlike autosomal trisomies, Turner's syndrome becomes *less* common with advancing age.
    (c) **True** This is an interesting association because the pre-eclampsia occurs early in pregnancy (16–20 weeks).
    (d) **False** Hypoglycaemia is a problem because of fetal hyperinsulinaemia.
    (e) **True** This usually occurs in a grand multiparous patient and there is uterine atony.

        **OB 2, 3, 5**

141 (a) **True** Long-acting thyroid stimulating antibodies may still be present.
    (b) **True** Nevertheless, careful monitoring is warranted because tachycardia may precede the development of bradycardia.
    (c) **True** This is due to the resulting amnionitis and pyrexia.
    (d) **True** Only fetal arrythmia will exceed this rate.
    (e) **True** A fast flat trace occurs in acute blood loss or chronic anaemia due to immune haemolytic disease.

        **OB 5**

142 Spontaneous pre-term labour:
  (a) Multiple pregnancy is the commonest cause
  (b) Is defined as labour before the 34th week
  (c) Does not tend to recur in subsequent pregnancies
  (d) Is the commonest cause of perinatal mortality
  (e) Is common in pre-eclampsia

143 Symptoms and signs of the onset of labour include:
  (a) Braxton Hicks contractions
  (b) Absent fetal movement
  (c) Shortening of the cervix
  (d) Dilatation of the cervix
  (e) Spinnbarkeit

144 Uterine contractions in labour:
  (a) Start at the cornu
  (b) Involve uterine muscle retraction
  (c) Are painful due to ischaemia
  (d) Are efficient at 5 mmHg
  (e) Are consciously controllable

145 Fetal monitoring in labour:
  (a) Shows the normal heart rate to be 120–160 beats/min
  (b) May involve checking the fetal pH
  (c) Is mandatory
  (d) Looks for beat to beat variations
  (e) Measures uterine activity and heart rate

146 Active management of the third stage:
  (a) Involves the Matthews Duncan method
  (b) May involve intravenous syntocinon
  (c) Increases the risk of needing a manual removal
  (d) Increases the chance of post-partum haemorrhage
  (e) Begins with delivery of the fetal trunk

142 **(a) False** Unexplained is by far the most common cause.
   **(b) False** It is defined as labour before the 37th week. However, no attempt is made to stop labour after the 34th or 35th week.
   **(c) False** A previous history of premature delivery is a strong risk factor for another premature delivery.
   **(d) True**
   **(e) False** However, early labour is often induced for this reason.

**OB 5**

143 **(a) False** These may be felt throughout pregnancy as painless, irregular contractions.
   **(b) False** Absence of fetal movements should always be regarded with suspicion.
   **(c) True** This is the earliest change in the latent phase of labour.
   **(d) True** This may be more difficult to determine in a multigravid woman as the cervical os may be 1 cm dilated in late pregnancy.
   **(e) False** This is a change in the cervical mucus seen at ovulation.

**OB 4**

144 **(a) True** Electrical traces show that the contraction wave starts near one or other cornu.
   **(b) True** When the contraction relaxes, some of the shortening of the fibres is maintained.
   **(c) True** The pain is analogous to the pain of myocardial ischaemia in coronary artery narrowing.
   **(d) False** Contractions are not palpable when less than 20 mmHg, and efficient contractions reach a pressure of 50 mmHg.
   **(e) False** Although the perception of pain may be altered by emotional state, contractions are not under conscious control.

**OB 4**

145 **(a) True**
   **(b) True** Fetal scalp blood samples for pH may be taken if there are abnormalities on the CTG tracing, or meconium-stained liquor.
   **(c) False** Low-risk normal mothers need intermittent ausculation only.
   **(d) True** Lack of beat-to-beat variation may indicate fetal distress.
   **(e) True** Both uterine activity and fetal heart rate may be measured either externally or internally.

**OB 5**

146 **(a) False** This is a description of the passive delivery of the placenta.
   **(b) True** Syntocinon is less likely to cause nausea and vomiting than ergometrine, and the intravenous route gives a quicker mode of action.
   **(c) True** There is a small risk that the contracting upper segment closes the cervix, trapping the placenta.
   **(d) False** The use of oxytocics and active management reduces the risk of PPH.
   **(e) False** It begins with an injection of an oxytocic agent with the delivery of the anterior shoulder.          **OB 4**

147 The second stage of labour:
  (a) Causes a transient bradycardia with contractions which are of little significance
  (b) Is less painful than the first
  (c) Ends with placental separation
  (d) Starts with pushing
  (e) Is shorter in multipara

148 The third stage of labour:
  (a) Starts early in the second stage
  (b) Ends with placental separation
  (c) Ends uterine activity
  (d) Generally involves >200 ml blood loss
  (e) Involves retraction of uterine muscle

149 The following predispose to primary post-partum haemorrhage:
  (a) Administration of prolonged or deep anaesthesia to the mother
  (b) Twin pregnancy
  (c) Oligohydramnios
  (d) Prolonged labour caused by mechanical difficulty
  (e) Hyperemesis gravidarum

150 Concerning third stage traumatic lesions:
  (a) Repair of a third degree perineal tear should not be attempted using only local anaesthesia
  (b) A second degree tear involves the perineal body and includes the anal sphincter
  (c) An extensive tear of the vagina can occur without a tear in the perineum
  (d) The symptoms of fistulae resulting from pressure necrosis during prolonged labour appear immediately after delivery
  (e) Fistulae resulting from direct trauma (e.g. during caesarean section or craniotomy) should not be repaired for 2–3 months

151 The following are contra-indications to intravenous beta-adrenergic stimulant therapy in obstetric practice:
  (a) Pre-term labour
  (b) Fetal distress in labour
  (c) Previous caesarean section
  (d) Asthma
  (e) Insulin-dependent diabetes

147 (a) **True** There are often decelerations due to head compression.
    (b) **True** Although the intensity of the contractions is greater, the positive action of pushing masks the severity of pain.
    (c) **False** It ends with delivery of the fetus.
    (d) **False**
    (e) **True** The second stage may be only a few minutes in multipara.

**OB 4**

148 (a) **False** It starts when the fetus has been delivered.
    (b) **False** It ends when the placenta and membranes have been completely delivered.
    (c) **False** Uterine retraction continues into the puerperium.
    (d) **False** Mean blood loss is <200 ml.
    (e) **True**

149 (a) **True** Anaesthesia, particularly the use of halothane, may cause uterine relaxation.
    (b) **True** Overdistension of the uterus predisposes to failure of retraction.
    (c) **False**
    (d) **True** Incoordinate uterine action occurs after prolonged labour.
    (e) **False** There is no such association.

**OB 5**

150 (a) **True** General or regional (i.e. spinal or epidural) anaesthesia should be used.
    (b) **False** Laceration of the anal sphincter places the tear into the category of the third degree.
    (c) **False** Such lacerations may cause considerable bleeding and be a cause of post-partum haemorrhage.
    (d) **False** The symptoms frequently do not appear for 10 days.
    (e) **False** Recognition, and immediate surgical repair, is the correct management.

**OB 5**

151 (a) **False** This is the primary indication for this therapy.
    (b) **False** Uterine contractions obstruct placental blood flow and it is the asphyxia, in an already compromised fetus, that causes distress. Abolition of contractions by beta-stimulant therapy is therefore beneficial while arranging measures for delivery.
    (c) **False**
    (d) **False** This is an indication for beta-adrenergic stimulant therapy. Cardiac disease, especially aortic and mitral stenosis, are contra-indications.
    (e) **True** The insulin requirement increases by about five times on this treatment and the disease becomes difficult to control. This effect is further aggravated if steroids are given to hasten fetal lung maturity.

**OB 5**

152 The following are absolute contra-indications to epidural analgesia:
  (a) Hypertrophic obstructive cardiomyopathy
  (b) Pilonidal sinus
  (c) Abruptio placentae
  (d) Pre-term labour
  (e) Twins

153 Syntocinon augmentation of labour:
  (a) Is more often required in multiparous patients
  (b) Aggravates fetal distress
  (c) May cause a prolonged hypertonic uterine contraction
  (d) May have to be reduced as labour progresses
  (e) May cause or aggravate neonatal jaundice

154 Fetal distress during the first stage of labour:
  (a) Always causes type II dips (late decelerations)
  (b) Can be diagnosed with a high degree of confidence if meconium is present
  (c) Is associated with an accumulation of lactic acid in the fetus
  (d) Should be treated with an infusion of bicarbonate
  (e) Can be helped by oxygen and glucose in the short term, while making preparations for caesarean section

152 **(a) True** In this condition, any reduction in end diastolic volume narrows the ventricular outflow tract and aggravates failure. The reduced left ventricular pressures will increase the shunt in Eisenmenger's syndrome and this is therefore also an absolute contra-indication. Other forms of heart disease may benefit from epidural analgesia because the increased cardiac output caused by pain and fright is diminished.

**(b) True** Any local sepsis will predispose to an epidural abscess.

**(c) True** (i) Shock is likely to be aggravated by abolishing protective vasoconstriction. (ii) Bleeding may occur into the epidural space as a result of consumptive coagulopathy.

**(d) False** By avoiding the use of drugs which inhibit respiration, this technique may be especially suited for premature labour.

**(e) False** Epidural analgesia is suitable for twin delivery and will allow a rapid delivery to be effected if fetal distress, cord prolapse or other complications occur after delivery of the first twin.

**OB 4**

153 **(a) False** Hypotonic inertia in the absence of disproportion is commoner in primiparous patients.

**(b) True** Uterine contractions always obstruct placental blood flow. They become stronger with syntocinon and the recovery phase between contractions is shortened.

**(c) True** This causes fetal distress, and may cause uterine rupture.

**(d) True** Labour is a self-perpetuating process and the dose may have to be reduced if contractions occur too frequently as this will cause fetal asphyxia.

**(e) True** This may be due in part to the antidiuretic effect of oxytocin causing red cells to swell and become less distensible. Such cells are more rapidly removed from the circulation.

**OB 5**

154 **(a) False** Although type II dips are often caused by fetal distress, other cardiotocograph changes, e.g. bradycardia, loss of beat-to-beat variation may indicate fetal distress. Only 35% of fetuses with type II dips are hypoxic at birth.

**(b) False** The passage of meconium due to vagal stimulation and contraction of the bowel may occur in fetal distress but the association is not strong.

**(c) True** Fetal distress is usually caused by hypoxia. This causes anaerobic metabolism and lactate accumulation.

**(d) False** Although the fetus is acidotic, bicarbonate is not helpful as it does not cross the placenta well. It also shifts the mother's oxygen dissociation curve to the left, which may further aggravate fetal hypoxia.

**(e) False** Oxygen is of benefit but glucose compounds lactate accumulation and hastens fetal death.

**OB 5**

155 The following predispose to fetal distress in labour:
   (a) The supine position
   (b) Pre-eclampsia
   (c) Renal disease
   (d) Lupus erythematosus
   (e) Pethidine administration

156 Prior to engagement of the fetal head:
   (a) The vertex may be visible at the vulva
   (b) A trial of forceps may be carried out provided that the vertex has passed the plane of the pelvic inlet
   (c) Three-fifths or more of the head are palpable abdominally
   (d) Induction of labour should not be carried out
   (e) Spontaneous labour is unlikely to start

157 Prolapse of the umbilical cord:
   (a) May occur while the membranes are still intact
   (b) Is a risk of induction of labour with prostaglandin pessaries
   (c) Has an incidence of 1% of labours
   (d) Is more common in singleton than in twin deliveries
   (e) Causes severe respiratory acidosis in the fetus

158 The occipito-posterior position:
   (a) In an example of a malpresentation
   (b) Usually turns to deliver as the occipito-anterior position
   (c) May proceed to deep transverse arrest
   (d) Is associated with a prolonged first stage
   (e) Is associated with a prolonged second stage

159 Hyperthyroidism in pregnancy:
   (a) Should be treated surgically rather than with carbimazole
   (b) May lead to neonatal hyperthyroidism even though the mother's disease is treated
   (c) Should not be treated with anti-thyroid drugs
   (d) Can be diagnosed by total T4 measurement
   (e) Is always associated with increased long-acting thyroid stimulator

155 **(a) True**  Pressure on the inferior vena cava diminishes venous return to the right side of the heart, causing hypotension and reduced placental blood flow.

   **(b) True** ⎤  Narrowing of the spiral arteries together with vasospasm diminish
   **(c) True** ⎦  placental blood flow.

   **(d) True**  Patients with the 'lupus anti-coagulant' develop microthrombi in the placental circulation.

   **(e) False**  This predisposes to poor respiratory effort after delivery.

**OB 5**

156 **(a) True**  This is unusual but possible, especially when **(i)** the head is highly moulded, and **(ii)** the pelvis is very shallow – this is seen particularly in the Negro pelvis.

   **(b) False**  This is still a high forceps and should not be carried out.

   **(c) True**

   **(d) False**  Provided the head is stably over the brim of the pelvis, induction with prostaglandins may be attempted.

   **(e) False**  In 60% of multiparous and 40% of primiparous patients the head does not engage prior to labour.

**OB 5**

157 **(a) False**  A cord below the presenting part but in an intact bag of membranes is a cord presentation.

   **(b) False**  It is a risk of surgical induction with a high presenting part or in the presence of hydramnios.

   **(c) False**  A more accurate figure would be 0.3%.

   **(d) False**  It is very common with the second twin, especially if the membranes rupture (or are ruptured) before contractions resume and the presenting part descends.

   **(e) True**  This is the initial effect of rapidly accumulating carbon dioxide. Later the hypoxia will lead to a superimposed metabolic acidosis.

**OB 8**

158 **(a) False**  It is a malposition. Breech and face are malpresentations.

   **(b) True**  This happens in about 80% of cases.

   **(c) True**  This happens when anterior rotation of the occiput is arrested in the transverse position.

   **(d) True**  Contractions are often less effective. The head tends to be deflexed and engage by the sub-occipito frontal (10 cm) diameter.

   **(e) True**  Rotation takes place in the late first and second stages.

**OB5**

159 **(a) True**

   **(b) True**  Long-acting thyroid-stimulating hormone is a gamma-globulin which may cross the placenta and give rise to fetal hyperthyroidism.

   **(c) False**  Although carbimazole and propylthiouracil cross the placenta, this may be an advantage if the fetus is hyperthyroid.

   **(d) False**  Total thyroxine is raised in pregnancy and free thyroxine levels or a suppressed TRH test are necessary for biochemical diagnosis.

   **(e) False**  Long-acting thyroid stimulator is only rarely present.

**OB 3**

160 Anaemia in pregnancy:
  (a) Is defined as haemoglobin of 10.0 g/dl or less
  (b) May be caused by haemodilution of pregnancy
  (c) May be caused by hookworm infestation
  (d) When megaloblastic, is usually due to $B_{12}$ deficiency
  (e) Is relatively common in multiple pregnancy

161 In iron deficiency anaemia in pregnancy:
  (a) Mean corpuscular haemoglobin content and mean corpuscular concentration are both low
  (b) Mean corpuscular volume (MCV) is raised
  (c) Blood transfusion is indicated if haemoglobin levels fall to below 9.0 g/dl
  (d) There is usually a chronic blood loss causing the anaemia
  (e) There is an increased risk of pre-eclampsia

162 In sickle-cell disorders:
  (a) There is failure of formation of the beta-chain of haemoglobin
  (b) The haemoglobin level rarely falls below 9.0 g/dl
  (c) There is a high incidence in Negroes and Asians
  (d) Iron deficiency is usual
  (e) Crisis is unlikely to occur with the trait

163 Diabetes mellitus in pregnancy is associated with the following:
  (a) Increased incidence of congenital defects
  (b) Increased insulin requirements
  (c) Increased risk of placental abruption
  (d) High incidence of vaginal Trichomonas infection
  (e) Fetal macrosomia

164 In acute pyelonephritis in pregnancy:
  (a) The left kidney is affected more often than the right
  (b) The temperature rarely exceeds 39°C
  (c) Antibiotics should be started before bacteriological results are available
  (d) The incidence of fetal growth retardation and pre-term labour is increased
  (e) Intravenous pyelography should be carried out promptly

160 **(a) False** It is defined as haemoglobin level of <11.0 g/dl. The anaemia is not necessarily pathological but may be physiological due to dilution.

**(b) True** The plasma volume may increase by 30% or more, resulting in a dilutional anaemia, despite an increase in red cell mass.

**(c) True** This is the commonest cause of anaemia in some parts of the world.

**(d) False** $B_{12}$ deficiency is very rare in pregnancy and megaloblastic anaemia is usually due to folic acid deficiency.

**(e) True** This is a result of dilution, and increased iron and folate requirements.

**OB 3**

161 **(a) True** This is a differentiating feature from beta-thalassaemia, where the MCH is low but the MCHC is normal.

**(b) False** The MCV is low, with hypochromasia.

**(c) False** Blood transfusion is only indicated if the patient is near term, and so there is insufficient time to raise the haemoglobin with iron therapy.

**(d) False** Inadequate dietary iron is the usual cause.

**(e) False** There is no relationship between anaemia and pre-eclampsia.

**OB 3**

162 **(a) False** It is thalassaemia that is caused by defective beta-chain formation. In sickle-cell haemoglobin there is alteration in the amino acid structure of the chain.

**(b) False** Severe anaemia may occur in sickle-cell disease.

**(c) False** There is a high incidence in Negroes, but not in Asians.

**(d) False** Iron stores are usually adequate.

**(e) True** The concentration of HbS is usually too low for sickling to occur.

**OB 3**

163 **(a) True** There is a considerable increased risk of congenital abnormalities, particularly sacral dysgenesis.

**(b) True** The insulin requirements frequently double.

**(c) False** Although the placenta is larger, there is no increased risk of abruption.

**(d) False** It is vaginal Candida infection which is associated with diabetes.

**(e) True** Poorly controlled diabetes leads to fetal macrosomia and risk of obstructed labour.

**OB 3**

164 **(a) False** The right kidney is affected more often than the left.

**(b) False** Fevers of 39.5°C and above are common, and often associated with rigors.

**(c) True** Vigorous treatment with antibiotics should be instituted promptly because of the risk of septicaemia and pre-term labour.

**(d) True** Fetal growth retardation is more likely if there is a background of chronic renal disease.

**(e) False** It is only indicated for recurrent attacks of unilateral pyelonephritis, and even then is usually deferred until 6 weeks post-partum.

**OB 3**

165 In cardiac disease in pregnancy:
    (a) Congenital heart disease is the commonest cause
    (b) Cardiac failure should not be treated with digoxin
    (c) Delivery should be by planned caesarean section
    (d) Cardiac surgery is absolutely contra-indicated
    (e) Ergometrine should be avoided in the third stage

166 Congenital malformations can be attributed to maternal infection with:
    (a) Poliomyelitis
    (b) Toxoplasmosis
    (c) Measles
    (d) Cytomegalovirus
    (e) Chicken pox

167 The following drugs are known to be teratogenic:
    (a) Phenobarbitone
    (b) Diazepam
    (c) Alpha-methyldopa
    (d) Erythromycin
    (e) Thiazide diuretics

168 During pregnancy, the following conditions are usually exacerbated:
    (a) Peptic ulcer
    (b) Multiple sclerosis
    (c) Meralgia parasthetica
    (d) Dental caries
    (e) Psoriasis

165 (a) **True** Fifty years ago, rheumatic heart disease caused 90% of valvular abnormalities, but this figure has now fallen to less than 50%.

(b) **False** Digoxin is perfectly safe in pregnancy, although its efficiency in some forms of cardiac disease is minimal (e.g. mitral stenosis unless atrial fibrillation is also present).

(c) **False** Caesarean section is only advised for obstetric reasons.

(d) **False** Cardiopulmonary bypass and open-heart surgery carries a considerable risk of fetal loss, but closed heart surgery may be carried out with reasonable safety.

(e) **True** Ergometrine, by causine an increase in blood pressure and venous return, may precipitate cardiac failure.

**OB 3**

166 (a) **False** Poliomyelitis may cause paralysis of the newborn if acquired within a few days of delivery, but not congenital malformations.

(b) **True** Blindness, hydrocephaly and mental deficiency have all been reported.

(c) **False**

(d) **True** Although the majority of babies are not affected, mental retardation and deafness may occur.

(e) **False** Congenital infection may however occur if the mother has chicken-pox shortly before delivery.

**OB3**

167 (a) **False** Phenytoin, which is often given with phenobarbitone for epilepsy, is occasionally associated with chondrodysplasia punctata but this is not an indication to stop the drug. Folate should be given with phenytoin.

(b) **False** Diazepam may cause loss of beat-to-beat variation of heart rate and respiratory depression in the neonate, but is not teratogenic.

(c) **False** This drug and beta-blockers are the most widely used for hypertension in pregnancy.

(d) **False** Erythromycin, penicillin and cephalosporins are safe in pregnancy. (Sulphonamides may aggravate neonatal jaundice, tetracyclines damage teeth and bones, aminoglycosides occasionally damage the VIIIth nerve and trimethoprim antagonizes folate and therefore provides a theoretical teratogenic risk.)

(e) **False** They may, however, aggravate neonatal thrombocytopenia.

**OB 2**

168 (a) **False** Gastric acidity is often reduced, and although reflux oesophagitis is common, peptic ulcers usually subside in pregnancy.

(b) **False** Relapse may occur after delivery.

(c) **True** This condition is caused by entrapment of the lateral cutaneous nerve of the thigh.

(d) **True** Gingivitis is common in pregnancy and this exacerbates dental caries.

(e) **False** The increase in cortisol levels often improves psoriasis.

**OB 2 & 3**

169 Asymptomatic bacteruria in early pregnancy:
   (a) Is found in at least 10% of women at booking
   (b) Is only regarded as significant when the bacterial count is more than $10^6$ organisms/ml
   (c) Leads in later pregnancy to pyelonephritis in 30% of cases
   (d) Should be treated if there is a previous history of symptomatic UTI
   (e) Is usually caused by *Streptococcus faecalis*

170 The following predispose to deep venous thrombosis:
   (a) Caesarean section
   (b) Antenatal bed rest
   (c) Breast feeding
   (d) Varicose veins
   (e) Pelvic infection

171 After delivery:
   (a) A vulvovaginal haematoma should not be incised for fear of causing an abscess
   (b) Third degree tear usually leads to rectal incontinence despite immediate suture
   (c) Bimanual compression is useful to expel a retained placenta
   (d) A much more concentrated oxytocin infusion may be administered than would ever be used in labour
   (e) Only one 0.5 mg ampoule of ergometrine may be administered within the first hour

172 The following organisms are recognized causes of puerperal pelvic sepsis:
   (a) *Escherichia coli*
   (b) *Haemolytic streptoccocus* (group A)
   (c) *Haemophilus influenzae*
   (d) *Clostridium welchii*
   (e) *Staphylococcus aureus*

173 Puerperal sepsis due to *Haemolytic streptococcus* (group A):
   (a) May cause rigors
   (b) Is the commonest cause of maternal mortality
   (c) Is likely to be caused by endogenous infection
   (d) Haemoglobinuria is usual
   (e) Is treated with tetracycline

**169 (a) False** The incidence is 3–6%.

**(b) False** $10^5$ organisms is usually significant and warrants treatment or further counts.

**(c) True** It is arguable whether the risk of developing pyelonephritis justifies treating all women with asymptomatic bacteruria.

**(d) True** It should definitiely be treated with antibiotics if there is a previous history of UTI.

**(e) False** *Escherichia coli* is the infective organism in 80% of cases.

**OB 3**

**170 (a) True** Abdominal delivery considerably increases the risk of thrombo-embolism.

**(b) True** If there are other risk factors (e.g. age, obesity), prophylactic anticoagulants should be considered.

**(c) False** Suppression of lactation with oestrogen predisposes to thrombosis.

**(d) False** Varicose veins increase the risk of *superficial* thrombophlebitis.

**(e) True** This applies to post-partum infection in maternity patients.

**OB 3**

**171 (a) False** If tense, painful or enlarging, it is best decompressed and the bleeding vessel ligated or oversown.

**(b) False** The prognosis is excellent with adequate repair.

**(c) False** A retained placenta should be removed manually. Bimanual compression is useful foratonic post-partum haemorrhage.

**(d) True** In the treatment of atonic post-partum haemorrhage, doses such as 50 units in 500 ml may be given at 30–60 drops/min without the danger of uterine rupture that exists before delivery.

**(e) False** A maximum of two 0.5 mg dosages may be given in the case of severe atonic post-partum haemorrhage.

**OB5**

**172 (a) True** This is an endogenous organism and a common cause of local infection of perineal and vaginal lacerations.

**(b) True** This is an exogenous organism and a cause of severe infection.

**(c) False**

**(d) True** Clostridial infection is extremely rare nowadays, but may occur when there has been much tissue damage.

**(e) True** *Staphylococcus aureus* is an increasing problem, especially because of development of resistant strains.

**OB 7**

**173 (a) True**

**(b) False** Puerperal sepsis is now an infrequent cause of maternal mortality.

**(c) False** The source of infection is likely to be from attendants.

**(d) False** This occurs in clostridial infection.

**(e) False** Penicillin is the treatment of choice.

**OB 7**

174 Breast feeding has the following advantages over bottle feeding:
   (a) Human milk contains more protein
   (b) Human milk contains more carbohydrate
   (c) There is a lower incidence of cot death in breast-fed infants
   (d) There is a lower incidence of atopic conditions
   (e) It needs to be given less frequently


175 Engorgement of the breasts in a lactating mother is treated by:
   (a) Stopping feeding for 24 h
   (b) Giving diuretics
   (c) Manual or mechanical expression
   (d) Discarding brassieres
   (e) Analgesics

176 In puerperal breast abscess:
   (a) Streptococci are the most common infecting organism
   (b) Suppression of lactation is advisable
   (c) Surgical drainage is rarely necessary
   (d) The whole breast is affected
   (e) Antibiotics should always be given


177 Small-for-dates babies are particularly liable to develop:
   (a) Hypoglycaemia
   (b) Hypothermia
   (c) Respiratory distress syndrome (RDS)
   (d) Anaemia
   (e) Pneumonia


178 Cephalhaematoma:
   (a) Is caused by oedema of the subcutaneous layers of the scalp
   (b) Should be treated by aspiration
   (c) Most commonly lies over the occipital bone
   (d) Does not vary in tension with crying
   (e) May result in ossification and asymmetry of the skull

179 Perinatal mortality:
   (a) Includes all stillbirths
   (b) Includes all neonatal deaths in the first month of life
   (c) Is increased in social classes 4 and 5
   (d) Is higher for mothers aged under 20 than aged over 35 years
   (e) Is principally caused by congenital abnormality, prematurity, and rhesus disease

174 **(a) False**  There is too much protein in cows' milk.
    **(b) True**
    **(c) True**  Cause and effect are unproven.
    **(d) True**  Cows' milk protein is a powerful antigenic stimulus.
    **(e) False**  If anything, bottle feeds may be given less frequently because larger volumes can be given.

**OB 6**

175 **(a) False**  Encouragement of the flow is important.
    **(b) False**  Diuretics are potentially harmful to the baby.
    **(c) True**  This may be the only way to relieve the discomfort.
    **(d) False**  Firm support is important.
    **(e) True**

**OB6**

176 **(a) False**  *Staphylococcus aureus* is the commonest organism.
    **(b) True**  In mastitis, temporary suspension of breast feeding may suffice, but if there is an abscess, cessation of lactation is invariably necessary.
    **(c) False**  It is always necessary once an abscess has occurred.
    **(d) False**  It is usually segmental.
    **(e) True**

**OB7**

177 **(a) True**  Depletion of glycogen stores has occurred *in utero*, so frequent feeding is necessary to prevent this complication.
    **(b) True**  The lack of subcutaneous fat impairs heat conservation.
    **(c) False**  Pre-term babies, not small-for-dates babies, develop RDS.
    **(d) False**  Pre-term babies are liable to anaemia.
    **(e) False**  Small-for-dates babies are not especially prone to infection.

**OB9**

178 **(a) False**  It is a subperiosteal haematoma.
    **(b) False**  This may lead to infection.
    **(c) False**  It is usually over the pareital bones.
    **(d) True**
    **(e) True**  More usually complete absorption occurs.

**OB 9**

179 **(a) True**
    **(b) False**  It includes neonatal deaths in the first week of life.
    **(c) True**
    **(d) False**  Both groups have an increased risk of perinatal mortality, but the >35 years group have a higher rate than the <20 years.
    **(e) False**  Congenital abnormality, prematurity and *hypoxia* are the causes accounting for 75% of perinatal deaths. Rhesus disease is now a rare cause.

**OB 11**

180 Respiratory distress syndrome (RDS):
  (a) Usually occurs in infants born before the 34th week of gestation
  (b) Is more common in caesarean section babies
  (c) Is more common in babies born to diabetic women
  (d) Leads to cyanosis
  (e) Is treated by giving 100% oxygen

181 Requirements for a newborn baby include:
  (a) 150 ml of fluid per kg body weight per 24 h
  (b) 110 calories per kg body weight per 24 h
  (c) A twice daily bath
  (d) In breast-fed babies, 20 min from each breast at each feed
  (e) 400 IU vitamin D per day

182 The following are thought to protect against hyaline membrane disease in the neonate:
  (a) Intra-uterine growth retardation
  (b) Severe pre-eclampsia
  (c) Heroin addiction
  (d) Prolonged rupture of the membranes
  (e) Diabetes

183 To avoid potential medico-legal problems in breech delivery:
  (a) All breeches should be delivered by caesarean section
  (b) The parents should be given the choice of mode of delivery
  (c) Ultrasound assessment of fetal size should be done
  (d) X-ray pelvimetry is advisable
  (e) An epidural anaesthetic should be used

184 Home confinement is a potential source of litigation because:
  (a) There are inadequate facilities
  (b) There are unskilled attendants
  (c) Doctors are reluctant to attend such a confinement
  (d) There may be delay in obtaining skilled medical help
  (e) No mechanism exists for proper selection of cases

180 **(a) True** After 34 weeks, the fetal lung is generally mature.
 **(b) False** Provided the baby is not pre-term, caesarean section does not predispose to this condition.
 **(c) True**
 **(d) True** This is due to shunting of blood through unventilated areas.
 **(e) False** Oxygen concentration should be kept to a minimum necessary to relieve cyanosis.

**OB 9**

181 **(a) True**
 **(b) False** 110 calories/kg body weight is all that is required.
 **(c) False** Too frequent bathing may remove the natural skin oils.
 **(d) False** Ten min is usually sufficient.
 **(e) True** Breast milk contains sufficient vitamin D, but artificial feeds may need addition of vitamin D.

**OB 6**

182 **(a) True**
 **(b) True** These conditions all stress the fetus and promote surfactant production.
 **(c) True**
 **(d) True**
 **(e) False** Surfactant production – in particular the important phosphatidylglycerol component – is retarded in this condition.

**OB 9**

183 **(a) False** Litigation may rise from caesarean section and its complications just as readily as from vaginal delivery.
 **(b) False** Explanation and information should be given to the patient, but a recommendation of mode of delivery should be given.
 **(c) True** Vaginal delivery of very large and very small breech babies is more hazardous so the size should be assessed.
 **(d) True** This is particularly so in a primigravid breech, and is usually carried out at 36 weeks gestation.
 **(e) False** Although there are advantages in good pain relief in the first stage of labour, these may be offset by the loss of bearing down sensation in the second stage.

**OB 10**

184 **(a) False** Only low-risk cases should be booked for home confinement.
 **(b) False** Health authorities have a statutory requirement to make available fully qualified midwives for the care of home confinements.
 **(c) False** General practitioners have a statutory duty to attend if called. Most districts have either an obstetric flying squad or a trained ambulance paramedic team to go out in an emergency.
 **(d) True** The time factor may be crucial in dealing with an emergency at home.
 **(e) False** General practitioners may advise on the suitability of a case for home confinement, and may refer to a consultant for his or her opinion. **OB 10**